She Fought On Her Knees

She Fought On Her Knees

Cover design by Alexys V. Wolf
Photo credit: Spencer Black
Interior design by Fiverr, Aalisha

Kindle Publishing Platform

Published in the United States of America

ISBN- 9781728775890

1. Personal Growth
2. Self-help

She Fought On Her Knees

My Story with Breast Implant Illness

Table of Contents:

Table of Contents:

This book is dedicated to breast implant illness awareness and to all the women currently battling this debilitating disease.

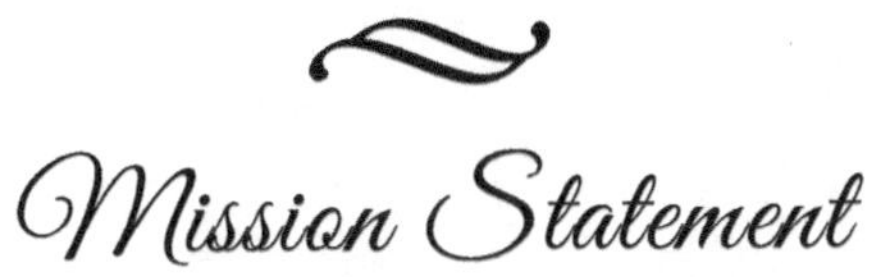

Mission Statement

My mission is to:

1. Teach people the love of God
2. Teach people how to love themselves as they are
3. Inform women about the perils of implants of any kind
4. Help women heal physically, mentally, emotionally and spiritually
5. Teach people how to pray through any given hardship

In my 46 years of life, I have learned that each day is a precious gift from God. It should not be taken for granted as no one is promised tomorrow. I've also learned that the life I was given is not just for me but it was given to me to help strengthen and encourage others. My purpose is to live a life guided by my faith in God and to lead by example in sharing truth. I plan to go about my mission by living a life fully surrendered to God in obedience to His Word while serving others.

Acknowledgments

First and foremost, I want to thank my Lord and Savior, Jesus Christ. Without whom, there would be no me to tell this story or encourage others.

Secondly, I thank my husband, Keith, and our kiddo's for never giving up hope, encouraging and enduring what, at times, seemed a losing battle.

Thirdly, I thank Alexys V. Wolf, my sister in Christ and editor, who put up with me at all times of the night emailing her edits to the book without complaining.

Last but not least, I thank the women with BII that have shared their stories in order to help other women battling this illness. We are a team. Thank you!

Introduction

Thank you for your interest in my journey scribed in the pages of *She Fought on Her Knees*. Whatever your reason is for purchasing the book, I pray you find the answers you seek. Matthew 7:7-8 reads, "Ask and it shall be given; seek, and ye shall find; knock, and it shall be opened unto you." Knowledge is power, power to make right decisions about your own body. Before we continue, let's be crystal clear in understanding that *breast implant illness* (BII) does not discriminate. It does not matter the reason someone had the implants due to mastectomy reconstruction, cosmetic, post-breast feeding mommy make-over, birth defect reconstruction, insecurity issues, etc., the illness is the same across the board and no one is exempt. This is the harsh reality. All will not heed to my warnings but, to the ones that listen, I say, "Amen".

By providing informational resources, my desire is to help other women avoid the same fate as mine. This is the place from whence this book was birthed. The sad part about this illness is that you, most likely, will not find answers or help from the medical community aside from surgical removal. With that being said, you must trust your body when it's telling you something is not right regardless of who may say otherwise. Women with breast implants (saline or silicone) have reported a garden variety of autoimmune diseases including rheumatoid arthritis, lupus and fibromyalgia combined with a host of varying ailments. While some studies concluded that breast implants do not cause autoimmune disease, most research focuses on women who only had implants a few months or years. Section II will offer numerous articles by various sources all pointing back to implants.

It is not my desire to have a debate, but it is my intention to make known to readers that breast implants have and will continue to make many, many women brutally ill. It happened to me and thousands upon thousands of other women. They made us all deathly ill. I am not the first and I won't be the last. Please note that both saline and silicone filled implants have an outer shell made of silicone which has known endocrine disruptors and can cause auto-immune symptoms and diseases. Like me, most women are not being informed of this fact. My personal recovery came only after I had my implants removed, otherwise known as *explanting*.

After stumbling upon a Facebook website and seeing all the women reporting the same symptoms as mine, I knew the implants were the cause of my sickness and needed to be removed immediately. That's when my husband and I began seeking doctors for explanting. All the women in the Facebook group were reporting being ill and were subsequently diagnosed with many ailments. Miraculously, they began feeling better and recovering once the implants were removed. That was the case with me as well. Coincidence? I think not.

Ultimately, the choice is yours regarding your own body. My prayer is that you educate yourself and choose wisely. In these pages you will find my story, how I had to pray on my knees so as to navigate my way through this whole ordeal and a few other stories as well. I had to fight my battle on my knees before Almighty God in hopes of discovering what was actually wrong with me and then find the correct solution. I wouldn't wish this battle on anyone.

This book is for anyone who has implants, knows someone with implants or desires to get them. If you fall in any of those categories, this book is a must read!

SECTION 1

My Journey

C H A P T E R   1

My Story's Beginning

I am a wife to the love of my life and the mother of the most amazing children. Prior to undergoing breast augmentation, I was like any normal working mother. I thought nothing of getting out of bed at 4:30am so as to make coffee and lunch for my husband, Keith. After getting up with him, I would lie back down for an hour or two. I would then get up again, assist my kids while they got ready for school, dropped them off and then took myself to work where I was a surgical tech for an oral surgeon. I have been in the dental field over 25 years.

I gave no thought to all the mundane things I would do on any given day such as handling surgical instruments during surgeries, holding things without pain and being able to move my fingers without incident or agonizing pain. I never thought about how long my days were because I had more than enough natural energy to get me through. I never considered the muscles in my body because I did not feel them. I gave no care to reading and being able to have clear vision to drive, cook, clean, work, etc. These things are normal everyday life for most people and so it was for me.

I was very healthy and lean. I exercised, ate healthily and did not drink alcohol or smoke cigarettes. I didn't take any medications other than a daily multivitamin and that was enough for me. The only surgeries I had prior to the illness were a tonsillectomy and appendix removal at an early age. I didn't need to visit a doctor of any kind on a regular basis. I was a perfectly healthy woman after having four children, all of whom I breastfed.

I was never an insecure woman and I never considered having breast augmentation because I was happy with my appearance. My husband didn't make me feel "less than" because I didn't have large breasts. However, because I had breastfed my children, I had lost fullness and desired to have that restored. My decision to go forward with augmentation was not for larger breasts but simply to get back what I had. Once I met with the surgeon, I moved forward.

On the day of the procedure, I was neither excited nor nervous; I had no emotions in either direction. It was simply something I had planned to do after childrearing. It was a "mommy make-over", so to speak. On the first post-op day, I had very minimal discomfort. Over the next couple days, I took about four of the pain pills the doctor had prescribed and needed no more after that. I followed all the instructions given to me so as to not cause damage.

As soon as I was released, I was back to my old self doing all the things status quo. It took three years to begin to experience signs of a problem. One by one, there were more and more symptoms but none, in and of themselves, caused alarm to me or my medical professionals. I had been given no warnings of the potential autoimmune risks and, to this day, doctors say there are none. Once they began to go into full swing, I began researching on my own so as to gain some clarity and help.

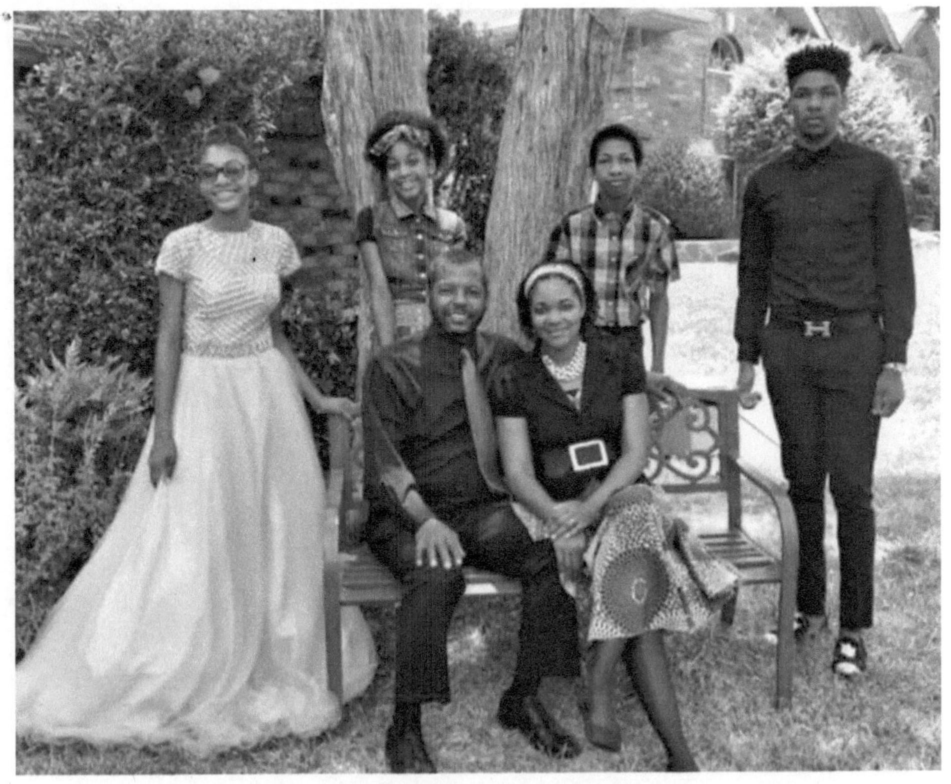

3 months after explanting

CHAPTER 2

The Slow Trickle of Symptoms

Symptoms of Implant Illness

Anxiety	Candida / yeast infections
Fatigue	Skin rashes / lesions
Joint pain	Visual disturbance
Muscle pain	Choking feeling
Insomnia	Ringing in ears
Brain fog	Headaches
Difficulty concentrating	Depression
Memory loss	Decreased libido
Limb numbness / tingling	Mood swings
Vertigo	Sharp pains in breast
Fever / chills	Weight gain
Muscle weakness	Food intolerance
Temperature intolerance	Swollen / tender lymph nodes
Sensitivity to light	Autoimmune symptoms or diagnosis
Sensitivity to sound	Chronic Fatigue Syndrome symptoms
Difficulty swallowing	Fibromyalgia symptoms
Hair loss	Inflammation
Dry skin / hair	Heart palpitations
Slow healing	Irritable bowel or bladder
Sinus infections	Shortness of breath
Recurrent illness	Night sweats

I had a total of 27 symptoms, two of which are not listed. The symptoms from BII came much earlier than I report because I didn't make the connection right away. I had my implants placed in 2013 by a very skilled surgeon via a referral from one of my employees. She was very pleased with her results and I was as well, at least initially. The total cost for my surgery was $6,500 which I paid out of pocket as the procedure was not covered under insurance.

As previously mentioned, my decision to get them did not stem from insecure body image, vanity or low self- esteem but rather to regain fullness after breast feeding. I thought to myself, "After all, implants are safe, right? Millions of women undergo this procedure each year for various reasons such as post-cancer mastectomy reconstruction, birth defects or cosmetic, and none of them ever get sick." Wrong! Although being made aware of basic complications that could arise from having implants including bleeding, scarring, capsular contracture, mild discomfort, implant rupture, and so on, I was not warned of the potential development of autoimmune disorders. Furthermore, I was never made aware that the outer shell of my implants was made of silicone.

Fast forward to 2017-2018, my health took a plunge exponentially for the worse; then came the weight gain. Looking back, it was gradual and came a little at a time. I went from weighing 125 lbs to 168 lbs in less than 3 years. I've been thin my entire life, very active, I ate healthily and I was a non-drinker and non-smoker. I could eat pretty much anything and it was hard for me to pick up any pounds. The inexplicable weight gain just kept coming and coming. No lifestyle changes had occurred except for the implants. No matter what I did, the weight would not budge. The doctor chalked it up to age-induced metabolism drop. Hmmmm…I don't think so. The worst of my symptoms were:

1. Passing out
2. Vision disturbance
3. Pain in left breast (not ruptured)
4. Extreme muscle and joint aches (diagnosed with fibromyalgia pre-explant)
5. Excessive weight gain

6. Brain fog (mimicked Alzheimer's)
7. Migraines
8. Night Sweats
9. Heart palpitations
10. Ringing in ears

Visual disturbance (2016)

I went from perfect vision to needing bifocals in what seemed like overnight. My eyesight began to deteriorate from weakened muscles. I went from 20/20 vision all my life to suddenly being diagnosed with a stigmatism. My vision was very blurry. I was in denial about it for quite some time after getting the glasses; I needed glasses but tried to convince myself I really didn't. Eventually the headaches started because I wasn't wearing them. I needed to wear them 24/7 so as to see.

The doctor stated that, with my age, it was not uncommon to have a sudden change in vision. I knew deep down this was not the case. I could see so much better with them but I could feel something in my eyes. I tried to describe the feeling; it was as though my eyes had a foreign substance in them. I couldn't quite articulate this to the doctor the way I really wanted. It was sort of like I had rheum (sleepers, eye discharge, gunk) in the lower part of my eye.

Extreme Fatigue (2017)

By the end of 2017, I started to notice I was waking up from a full night's sleep still feeling tired. Around the time of my cycles, I also noticed I was even more fatigued and lethargic to the point of not wanting get out of the bed. By this time, I was calling it a night around 8-8:30. I chalked this up to age and my body taking on a new vibe because I was getting older. As you can guess, that was not what was happening.

Weakening of My Muscles and Hernia Surgery (2017)

One morning while getting ready for work, a sudden sharp pain hit me in my lower groin area. After hollering in pain, I began to regurgitate and ball into a fetal position. I was home alone so I called Keith and he rushed home. I called in sick to work and headed to the emergency room. It was a hernia which had popped out. They didn't fix it there; they merely gave me antibiotics and pain meds. The next day I consulted with another doctor that told me she did not see a hernia on the x-rays. I told her I could feel it and that my right groin area was never like that before this incident. She still said she could not see it on the x-rays and would do exploratory surgery. Four days later, I had the surgery to repair the damage yet still had not linked it to the implants. After waking from the surgery, she stated, "You were right, you did have a hernia." That was in November 2017.

Chronic Muscle and Joint Pain (2017/2018)

Severe muscle and joint pain was one of my worst symptoms. Every joint in my body ached day and night without relief. The initial point of pain started with my right middle finger locking. We have a two-story home and I was unable to go up the stairs without stopping every three steps because I was in agony. I hurt everywhere. Soon I stopped going up the stairs just to avoid the pain. Every morning before I drove our youngest two kids to school, I needed my daughter to put my ankle zip-up boots on me because I could not bend down to do it myself. I left them unzipped because I knew that, after returning home, I would not be able to get them off. The muscle and joint aches continued and I still have issues with it today but it's bearable. I was also diagnosed with fibromyalgia and arthritis. The arthritis diagnosis came after my implants were removed.

Because I worked in oral surgery passing sharp instruments back and forth using repetitive motions, the hand specialist associated the pain and stiffness as work related. I wore a hand and finger splint for some time but, when there was no relief, I began to receive steroid injections. That worked like a charm but only lasted for about three months. After the second injection, I opted not to continue them because they were thinning my skin.

The specialist suggested surgery to correct the trigger finger permanently so I followed his advice. I had corrective surgery January 2018 and all went well. I was still not thinking this could possibly have something to do with my breast implants. After the surgery, my finger never locked again; however, the pain was still there. By this time, it was not just my one finger that had pain, it was both hands. Every single joint in my hands ached constantly. It was just a matter of time that the muscles in my hands began to become affected by my illness.

During the day, I would also have bouts of hand weakening. This caused me alarm as I felt very uncomfortable handling sharp instruments. This also came with episodes of dizziness unrelated to the trigger finger. At that point, I was not fit to assist anyone during any surgeries and informed the doctor I needed some time off for my own surgery. She was very obliging. That time off turned into not returning to work at all due to more complications of BII.

Brain Fog 2017-2018

I had brain fog so badly that I literally thought I had Alzheimer's disease at the age of 43; either that or brain damage! I can laugh at it now but it wasn't funny then, not one bit. Many times I just wanted to cry out of frustration. I've always been book-smart, but it had me questioning myself; I felt stupid and embarrassed. One day my co-worker asked me to do a task. I totally forgot what she asked me so, when she followed up with me hours later, she said, "Angelia, did you?" I confessed I didn't remember her asking me. I didn't remember what she asked me even when she said it again so as to refresh my memory. Of course I apologized and felt defeated as it really bothered me.

Another time I was at home and had this sudden urge to go somewhere. I hurriedly grabbed my purse and keys and got in the car. I drove about four blocks from my home and totally forgot where it was I wanted to go or what I had intended to do. I pulled into Walgreens (it was closest) and I sat there frustrated and unable to remember why and where I was going. This incident frustrated me so badly that I texted my husband afterwards and had a good cry. To this day, I cannot remember the purpose of getting into the vehicle. I can't count how many times I misplaced my keys on any given day and numerous times over and over. There are many, many other incidents such as this and, yes, it did start to wear down my confidence. I felt like something was really wrong with me and it was.

Tingling and Pain in Hands and Feet (2016-2018)

As previously mentioned, I had surgery on my right hand to correct finger locking and pain. The surgery was a success; however, I still had pain in my right hand. I was diagnosed with fibromyalgia and I had arthritis in both hands. I was referred to a rheumatologist and from there a neurologist. I was prescribed pain medicine, vitamin D and a muscle relaxer. The vitamin D was for a week only. I tried the pain meds and they didn't work. I soon realized the best relief was the muscle relaxer so that's all I took. With taking the muscle relaxers, I also noticed that within four days of taking them the tingling in both my hands went away. I'm currently taking the muscle relaxer and a one-a-day women's vitamin.

Passing out (2018)

My first episode of passing out was at my breast implant surgeon's office while waiting for a consultation. It happened again at home one night while getting up to go to the kitchen. It was so bad an ambulance was required to take me to the hospital. I remember none of the last episode as my family had to tell me about it. I woke up very frightened for my husband and kids. By the last episode, I had already been approved by my insurance company for the explants. I was waiting for my surgery date which was March 21st 2018.

CHAPTER 3

Stumbling Upon BII

It was getting very expensive as well as frustrating going to doctor after doctor to no avail. None of my blood work (like many other women) showed any waving red flags. Nevertheless, I was still sick and getting worse every day. It got so bad that I was practically bedridden given the intensity of the pain. The joint and muscle aches were constant with no relief at all. I finally ran across a doctor who believed in the existence and validity of BII so I went for a consultation. He explained that I was not the only one going through this (as I already deduced). He then told me of the many other women who suffered almost the exact same symptoms as mine. He also stated that nearly 99% of the women that had their implants removed saw improvement almost immediately; that the majority of the women who had them removed said the symptoms improved 60-100%.

On the Facebook group, the women who testified with their stories said that, post-explant, most had a full recovery. Many of the full recovery stories were not immediate but took 3-6 months. They also stated they had to detox their bodies after explanting so as to rid their bodies of the toxins. Many also suffered with leaky gut due to their compromised immune systems from the toxins. This had to be addressed after explanting with clean eating, medications, etc.

Finding the link between being sick and my implants did not come from a doctor. It came from my extensive search on the internet. I happened to stumble upon the Facebook group "Breast Implant Illness, Healing and Awareness by Nicole". This was the light bulb moment for me upon seeing the thousands of other women in this group who mentioned the same exact symptoms I was having. I had been told by medical professionals there was no scientific data to prove it was the implants. After reading their stories I knew they were suffering the same as I; they were 100% my same story just different people. After going from doctor to doctor and getting negative test result after negative test result, my husband and I finally decided to get the things out. I explanted on March 21st 2018 and it has proven to be one of the wisest decisions of my life. To date, I am about 99.9% healed. Praise the Lord! I finally found that for which I was searching and it turned out to be right. It was a no-brainer for me to have those toxic bags removed from my body.

It is an absolute tragedy that women such as me have to suffer in silence feeling as though there is no hope for recovery. For many women, they can easily go into a very dark place with feeling as though they are crazy, as though it's "all in my head". This is a horrific place to be, especially when the doctors and/or family members are echoing those sentiments. There is absolutely no possible way to fully express the depth of sensations of inadequacy, failure, hopelessness, exhaustion, frustration or altogether no reason to continue living. Because I had a great support system, I was surprised at some of the emotions I felt. Husbands have abandoned their wives because they don't understand what's happening to them and have no desire to help them get relief. I had help but still felt many dark emotions I could not have predicted.

Countless women are scorned mercilessly by those who are supposed to love them. Their husbands buckle under the pressure of not knowing what to do with their wives. Many women barely have enough energy or strength to get out of bed, much less enough go to work or properly care for their family. Because of BII, whole families have fallen apart. I know of newlyweds who, when they needed to explant, their husband left them before the ink on the marriage certificate was dry. Some men complain to their sickly wives that they look better with the implants and attempt to convince them they need to keep them. Women have been committed to insane asylums for less. Women suffering from BII who don't understand what they feel or why they feel it are committed to psychiatrists and prescribed antidepressants simply because they haven't gotten a proper diagnosis. It may sound farfetched but, I assure you, it is truth and it simply should not be.

CHAPTER 4

My Husband's Perspective

I would say that, initially, I didn't think her illness was due to breast implants and I really didn't understand her level of pain and suffering she was enduring on a daily basis. It wasn't until she started fainting and complaining about her vision that I started taking it seriously. It wasn't that I didn't take her seriously before but I genuinely didn't understand what was going on. I didn't see the connection between the symptoms and the implants; I felt strongly it was something else. It was Angelia who really educated me on the issues of having breast implants and, once she did, I started doing my own research and really seeing where other people were having the same health issues. I was praying about it and her condition for God to reveal what was going on so we could find help.

I know our experiences with the doctors didn't start out too well. It's crucial that you find the right doctor, one that believes in breast implant illness so as to provide the best service. It was pretty frightening and scary for me to see my wife go through this not knowing what was going on. Once we concluded it was coming from the implants, it was a relief. Finally we had something to point to and be able to correct the problems. If I could say one thing to another man whose wife is going through this, it would be to really listen to your wife; believe what they are saying and support them. It's one thing to hear a doctor say that it's in your head but it's another to hear it from your spouse. Although I never believed it was in her head, I was agitated because we couldn't get an answer from anyone.

The fainting was the most frightening for me because thoughts of losing her started entering my mind. It was hard for me to deal with because I did not want my mind to go there. I didn't want to display my fears in front of her. Once we found out there was a cure which was implant removal (explanting), that was my prayer being answered because I knew it could be fixed. It was a blessing to know our insurance would cover the removal; most insurance companies will not cover this surgery for most women. It's definitely something for which we both are grateful. I can say today that she is back to herself. She isn't fainting. Her energy is restored. Her vision is better. Most things returned to normal.

Once Angelia went through the surgery, she almost immediately began recovery. Her vision started coming back and other pains immediately diminished. The most frustrating part for me is that, with all the evidence of improvement from so many women post-explant, the doctors are not investing time and energy needed with the illness. I'm not convinced women really understand the risk when they are considering having breast implants or being properly informed. I know she and I have different views than the doctors when they say that there is absolutely no evidence of implant illness. They say they have no source or scientific evidence to prove otherwise.

There is a lot of evidence out there. When you listen to all the stories of recovery post-explant via Facebook and social media, it doesn't make sense that the stance of doctors and scientist are dismissive. It's a shame because this illness is all too real and the recovery from removal is real. I cannot say whether or not I would be skeptical if someone other than my wife told me their story or if I didn't live through it myself and witness it firsthand. Regardless, living through it with her has made me a firm believer. I feel terrible for women who know what's causing them to be sick yet do not have the means to have them removed. I genuinely believe insurance companies should take a hard look when it comes to explanting because it could be a matter of life and death.

We kept her illness from the kids as long as we could until we found out there was something that could be done. We did not want to place unnecessary strain on them; however, once there were obvious changes in her appearance and needing help with everyday tasks such as getting out of bed, we couldn't hide it any longer. Things like putting on her shoes, taking off her shirts over her head, zipping boots and medial daily tasks became too much for her to bear. I vividly recall having to help her put on her shoes and clothes and it sincerely scared me. I didn't know where it was going and I was trying not to show too much concern as I didn't want to escalate any more fear in her. It really did frighten me and that's just keeping it real. I experienced this firsthand day in and day out. We had to fight as a team and we did. She fought on her knees and so did I.

Prayer and persistence in seeking answers for a cure was our only route to her recovery. There is nothing greater than being able to place all problems, doubts and darkness onto a God who hears and responds. Faith was our guiding light and strong fortress through it all. My wife is the strongest woman I have ever known and I cannot imagine life without her. I thank God regularly for her life and her recovery. It's a huge answer to prayer.

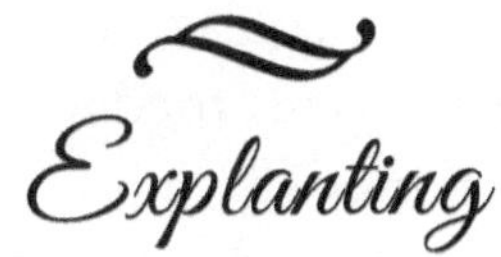

CHAPTER 5

Explanting

My explant surgery cost around $12,000 and the surgery went very well. The surgeon was extremely skilled and was able to take the entire capsule out in en bloc form. He also provided photos of the implants and capsule. As a family, it took a toll on us mentally, physically and financially but we made it through with love and prayer. As previously stated, I've heard numerous stories where husbands and family members were not understanding or supportive. As for those women, my heart breaks.

My Detox Regimen:

The first day after surgery, I stayed in the bed. I felt so good I wanted to do everything! I noticed immediately that some symptoms went away such as:

1. vision cleared
2. eye redness went away
3. dead feeling was gone
4. increased energy

I still had the drains from surgery but they didn't stop me. I followed the doctor's orders of no reaching, heavy lifting, etc. I ordered a liquid from Amazon so as to aid in cleansing my gut which had been damaged by the illness. Leaky gut is no joke! The supplement I used is (green) black walnut wormwood complex herbal supplement. The brand name I used was "Now." I took two droplets of this a day mixed with orange juice. Together it tasted like grapefruit juice so the taste wasn't too bad at all. I was also on an antibiotic and was sent home with a prescription for pain meds. I took the entire antibiotic and about eight of the pain meds.

I didn't experience much pain after the surgery but everyone is different; I didn't need much down-time. Again, everyone is different so don't get discouraged if it takes you longer to heal post-surgery. Allow your body to heal at the pace needed without comparing yourself to others. I also drank lots of water and ate organic bone broth for the first week after surgery. Also, I only ate organically after I was finished with the bone broth. I had no sugar for one month after surgery and I ate raw garlic. That garlic thing was…ahem…HOT! I washed it, peeled it, cut it into small pieces, chewed and swallowed it with some juice. I ate one small, fresh garlic a day along with four fresh cloves. I chewed it finely and followed it with some orange juice.

I began lightly walking outside after two weeks and jogging four weeks after surgery. I also did ultraviolet sauna so as to sweat out the toxins; I went twice in a month. All my symptoms were completely gone. Only one symptom returned about six months after surgery which was the hand pain and the joints ached daily. Please see other BII groups for detox regimes. I had massage treatments as well for my aching muscles and joints.

I went from having 20/20 vision to bifocals to later needing a stronger prescription in less than eight months. Post-op, I didn't need glasses at all! My vision returned to normal immediately after I awoke from anesthesia. I am truly amazed at the expediency of my recovery. I am dumbfounded by the negligence of the medical industry where implants are concerned. There is absolutely no reason for this other than, with public knowledge, money would be taken out of the hands of greedy manufacturers and doctors. The more we know, the better and more informed decisions we can make about our own bodies.

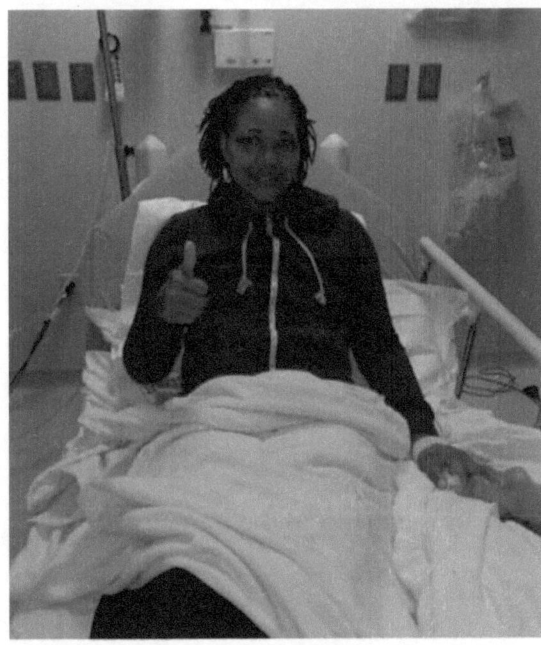

just after the surgery

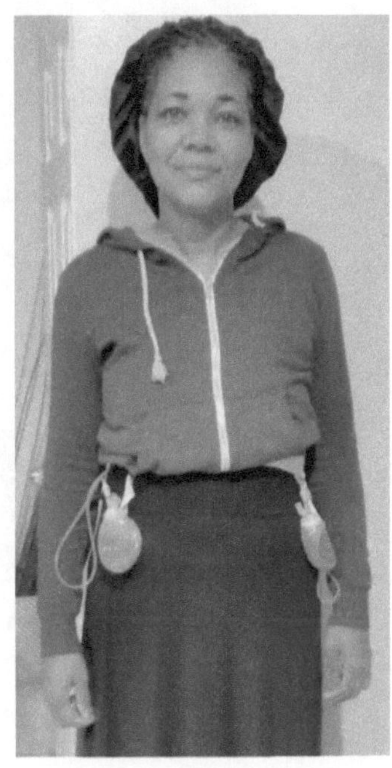

day after surgery with drains

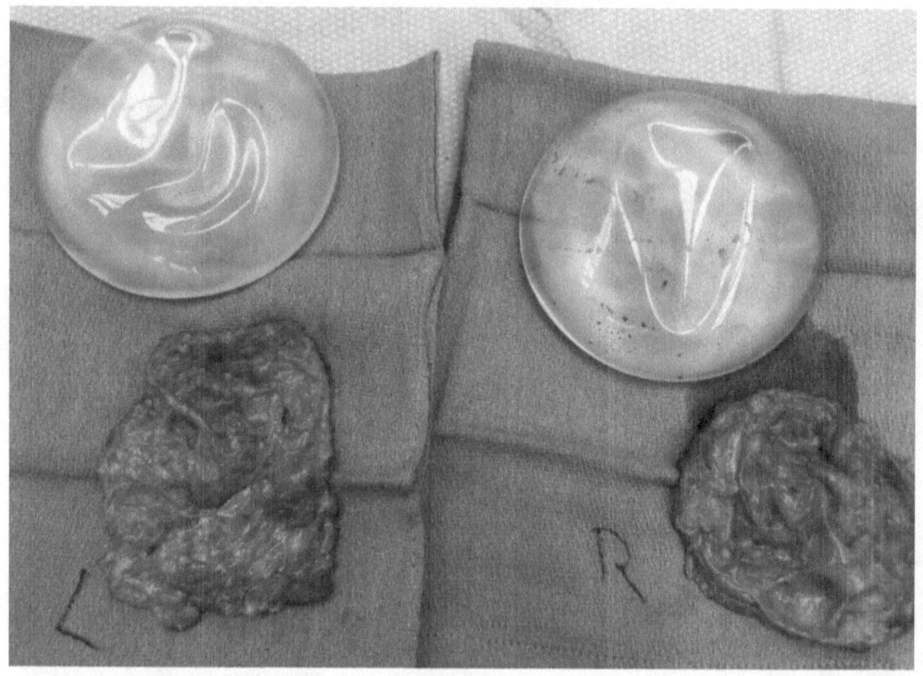

implants with capsules that formed around the implants

CHAPTER 6

Dealing with My Anger

"But if you do not forgive others, then your Father will not forgive your transgressions (Matthew 6:15)."

"Judge not, and you will not be judged; condemn not, and you will not be condemned; forgive, and you will be forgiven (Juke 6:37)."

Initially, I started this book from a point of anger and hurt. Anger because, after all, implants were supposed to be safe, right? They were supposed to help people, not harm them. They were supposed to restore people's confidence and mend broken bodies, not be a cash-cow so as to line the deep pockets of the surgeons. With my story, something went very wrong. They didn't restore; they stole my quality of life. The implants didn't help, they harmed. They were not safe but very toxic. I was never warned of any of these potential outcomes. I was never told there was a possibility of developing an autoimmune disease.

With that being said, surely you can understand my desire to write from a place of anger so as to let my offenders (surgeons and medical staff) know I was angry, mad, disgusted, hurt, and more. Nevertheless, after praying about it, "forgive" is what the Lord prompted me to do. After praying, my desire was no longer to write from a hurting, angry heart. Does that mean that I was not angry? Absolutely not, but I did not let anger remain. There I was with an almost completed book and all I heard was "forgive". That wasn't the message I wanted to hear at that moment! Forgiving "those people" translated into me being forgiven by the God whom I call Father. Through extending forgiveness and releasing those whom I felt owed me something, I was equipped to take back my power and peace. After all, forgiveness is not for the offender but for the person offended.

I took my power back, power which I had unwittingly given others by holding a grudge; bitterness was about to eat me alive from the inside out. As it so happens, my toxic heart was just as bad as the toxic implants I had removed seven months prior. Was I a victim of medical negligence, absolutely, and there's no denying it. Did I have every right to be angry about that? Indeed I did but, as a believer in Christ Jesus, I am commanded to forgive and I did. The Lord has turned my medical mess into a message. I am now able to reach others so they may avoid the same nightmare I and thousands of other women have endured and are still battling. I pray that something I say in this book will bless and touch many in a special way, especially the part about forgiveness. I now am quicker than ever to forgive versus holding a grudge. I valued this truth in one of my darkest moments. Forgiveness was a part of my healing. It is much harder for a physical body to heal when its life source is bitter and angry. An unforgiving heart is vile and as a growing cancer.

You're probably thinking right now, "Is she serious?! Forgive who?" I can only speak for myself because I speak from my faith. This was one of the most important parts of the healing process for me. Forgiving those who knowingly and unknowingly harmed me was paramount to my healing process. My Aunt Clarice Coleman says, "Unforgiveness is like drinking poison and expecting the other person to die." There is no value in unforgiveness.

For those reading this that do not walk with God through His Son, Jesus, this won't make any real sense to you. Notwithstanding, for those who do, Hebrews 12:15 states, nay, commands, "See to it that no one comes short of the grace of God; that no root of bitterness springing up causes trouble, and by it many be defiled." Unforgiveness and bitterness are nothing short of intangible toxic poison. When they run through someone's veins, they destroy a person slowly and surely. "See to it" is not a suggestion from God but a command. We must all "see to bitterness and unforgiveness so that they are not allowed to take root and contaminate you or those around you.

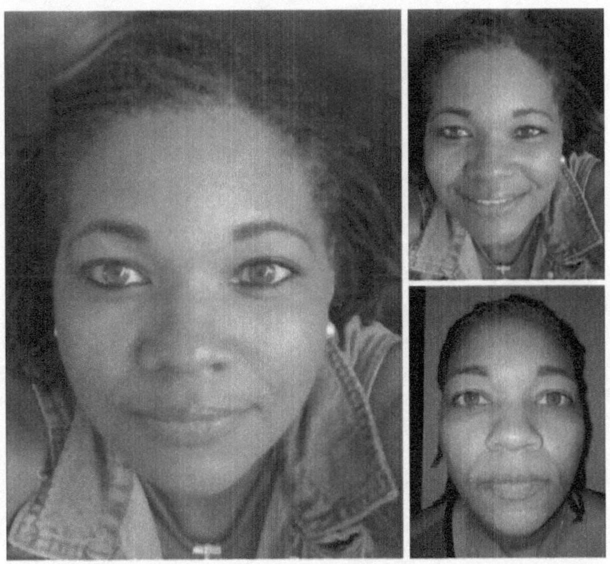

day before surgery and one week after

C H A P T E R 7

Testing of Faith

"God is our refuge and strength, an ever-present help in trouble. Therefore we will not fear…(Psalm 46:1-3)."

"And the God of all grace, who called you to His eternal glory in Christ, after you have suffered a little while, will Himself restore you and make you strong, firm and steadfast (I Peter 5:10)."

Just about all my life I have been a person of faith in our Lord Jesus Christ. I was raised in church and I believed at a young age. I always purposed to put God first and live a life in accordance to the Spirit of God. That being said, I must confess, this struggle was unlike anything I have ever experienced. This situation of BII and autoimmune issues put my faith to the test to say the very least! I had never known such pain and agony in my body. The fact that I had no idea why it was happening added insult to injury. I had heard of autoimmune disease before but had no clue what it was all about until my body was riddled with it.

I can remember purposing to hide my true level of pain from Keith and the kids because I did not want to worry them needlessly. After months of struggling, things went from bad to worse. Seeking

29

answers from doctors left me more frustrated than ever. I had medicines and surgeries so as to correct the situation to no avail. Things would help temporarily but, inevitably, the pain would come right back. I can honestly say that, through it all, never once did I question God about my situation from a stance of blaming Him. Regardless of whether or not He healed and restored my health, I was determined to use my testimony so as to encourage others. I was angry at the pain. I was angry I wasn't getting relief. I was angry I would eventually have to change jobs since I could no longer steadily hold sharp instruments. My life seemed to be crumbling and my body was attacking itself.

All I could do was get on my knees and pray to Almighty God for direction, answers and resolution. I didn't know if this would be my early demise or if I would have to live a long and agonizing life; I simply didn't know what was going on. I clung to the Word of God even when I didn't want to or didn't feel like it. I grabbed hold of all God's infallible promises and held tightly until I began to see them come to fruition in my life. This testing of faith was the most difficult challenge of my life and I am altogether grateful for the opportunity to now be able to say that I came through. And not just that; I came through stronger in my faith and I see God's hand in it all. Because of this journey, I'm now able to aid others in their journey with BII, low self-esteem, body shaming, issues with placing their value on their physical body, and other misconceptions about themselves which would lead them to a bad decision of breast implants.

The testing of my faith led me to understand God in a much more personal, intimate and significant way. It's difficult to have true compassion when you have never experienced any real suffering. Some may disagree with me but look around the body of Christ. People who have never gone through a major ordeal of any kind have much less patience and compassion for those who are in crisis. It's easy to become calloused, critical and judgmental because, after all, "I love Jesus and it isn't happening to me." Very well-meaning Christians who have not endured trials are quick to (even if they don't say it) pass judgment assuming everyone in a tribulation must have hidden sin or a severe lack of faith. It's true. People are really like this within the confines of the body of Christ and it should not be true.

Once any of us really have our faith tested on a level no one would ever seek, when we come out, we will either walk away from God in bitterness and anger or we will see God for the Savior and Sovereign He is. For the latter, we will begin to extend loving compassion like never before. The testing of faith is mandatory for all who call upon the name of Jesus, not just the strong. In fact, such testing will reveal who we really are underneath the clean-cut church façade. I am truly thankful to God for taking me through this because it has deepened my walk of faith, my relationship with the Lord, and my understanding of how much He loves us in our frailty of life.

This experience has opened my eyes to how precious are life and good health. I didn't mean to but I recognize that, within myself, I took it all for granted. I never thought about what a blessing it was to simply be able to get out of bed pain free or to cook, work, and care for my family until this came about. What a time of revelation! No one wants to go through pain, suffering, agony, cluelessness, etc. but, on the other side, we are much better for it.

Feeling my health return was a most extraordinary, exuberating, enlightening blessing from God! Just being able to return to a normal existence was liberating. I appreciate breathing more than ever. I value the little things which I never did before. I thank God daily for my restoration on every level. Fighting on my knees equipped me to stand firmly in God's promises.

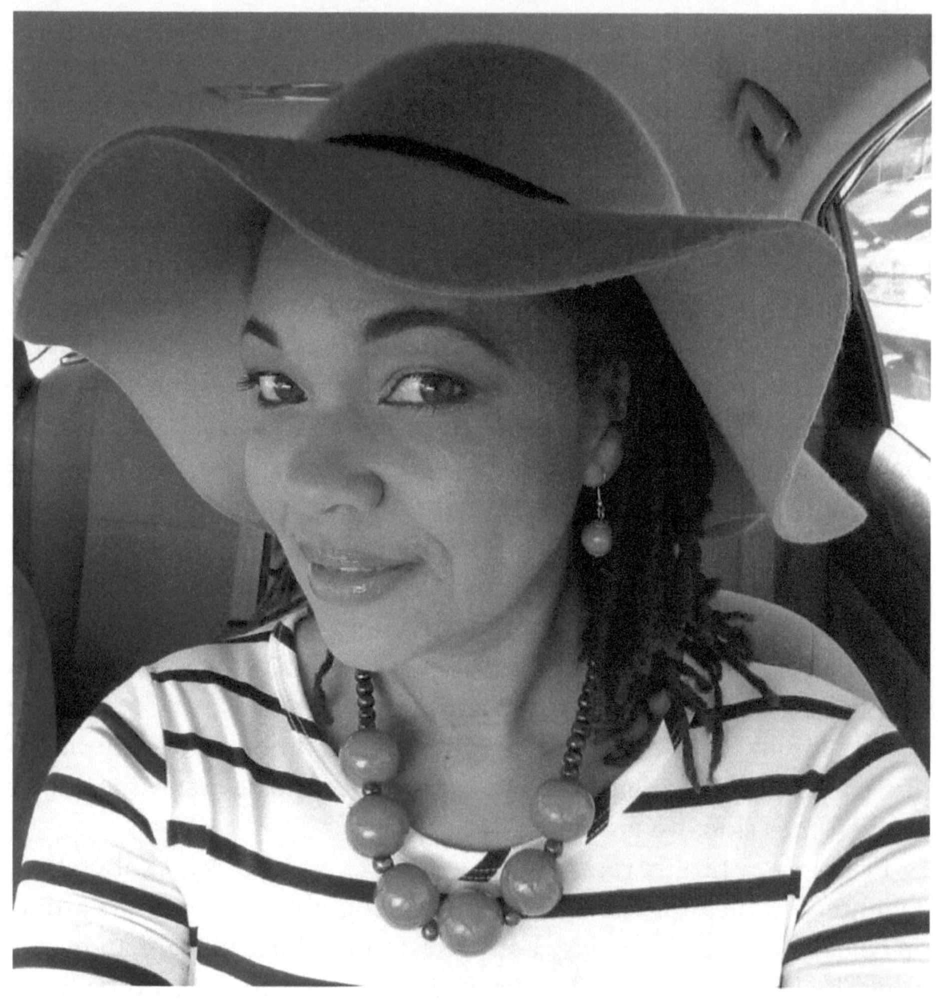

one year post-explant

Clinical Perspective of BJJ

C H A P T E R   1

Autoimmune Symptoms and

"Breast Implant Illness"

This information was taken directly from:
https://breastimplantinfo.org/autoimmune-symptoms-breast-im-plants/?gclid=EAIaIQobChMIlp_Im7rD4QIVSeDICh-23BA5IEAAYAiAAEgL_NvD_BwE

NATIONAL CENTER FOR HEALTH RESEARCH *presents*:

Autoimmune Symptoms and "Breast Implant Illness"

Breast implant companies were required to complete safety studies before they could sell their implants in the United States. Although the Food and Drug Administration (FDA) approved breast implants, they admitted that "studies would need to be larger and longer" to find out if implants could cause the kinds of symptoms and diseases many women were reporting.[1] Those symptoms and diseases are often referred to as "breast implant illness" by the women, although that is not a medical diagnosis.

Since many women reported problems with autoimmune or connective tissue disorder symptoms such as joint pain and fatigue, breast implant companies did_not study the safety of implants in women who had a family history or personal history of autoimmune disease before getting implants. They intentionally excluded those women because they were concerned that those women might be more likely to have health problems from the implants. Breast implant companies recognize this as a shortcoming of their studies. For example, this is what Mentor says in their label for MemoryGel® implants:[2]

"Safety and effectiveness have not been established in patients with the following:

- *Autoimmune diseases (for example, lupus and scleroderma)…"*

Unfortunately, most physicians and most women considering implants are unaware of that warning.

What Is Autoimmune Disease?

Autoimmune disease is a condition where immune cells attack your body. Immune cells usually help our bodies fight off infections and foreign substances. However, these immune cells see silicone as a foreign substance, and that can cause the body to start an immune response.

In some cases, the immune system launches a big enough attack that it starts attacking the body. This could lead to symptoms like joint pain, fatigue, mental confusion, dry eyes, and hair loss. Some women with breast implants report a wide range of symptoms that do not fit into one specific condition. Over time, some women develop a pattern of symptoms that are diagnosed as lupus, scleroderma, fibromyalgia, or other conditions. Autoimmune diseases can target specific organs, like the brain or liver. They can also involve many tissues, like muscles or blood.[3]

It is important to know that not all people who get breast implants develop immune problems. Those who develop autoimmune symptoms may have other risk factors, such as allergies or a family history of autoimmune disease.[4] In addition, women who already had autoimmune symptoms can get worse symptoms or new symptoms after getting breast implants. Certain genes may also increase the chances of developing autoimmune diseases or symptoms, sometimes as a reaction to silicone or other exposures. In addition, women who already had autoimmune symptoms can get worse symptoms or new symptoms after getting breast implants.

How "Good" Is the Evidence?

There is conflicting evidence from studies that examined whether breast implants cause autoimmune disease or symptoms. Most studies were funded by implant companies or plastic surgery associations, and they tend to focus on narrowly defined diagnoses, with numerous studies based on hospital records rather than medical records. However, many women with breast implants have reported the same complaints over the last few decades, and many women report that their symptoms greatly improved or completely disappeared after their implants were removed. A study published in 2013, by researchers in the Netherlands, found that 69% of women with autoimmune symptoms who had their implants removed experienced reduction in symptoms and almost 20% experienced full recoveries after explanation. [5]

In 2001, FDA scientists reported that women whose ruptured breast implants leaked silicone outside the scar tissue surrounding the implant were significantly more likely to have been diagnosed with fibromyalgia (a painful soft-tissue disease), pulmonary fibrosis, and connective-tissue diseases such as dermatomyositis.[6] Fibromyalgia is a disorder that causes widespread pain in the body as well as fatigue. Little is known about how fibromyalgia develops, but researchers think it is an immune system problem.

In 2004, scientists from the National Cancer Institute reported that women with breast implants were more likely to have autoimmune symptoms. However, because symptoms were self-reported, the scientists concluded that more research was needed to determine if breast implants caused specific symptoms or diseases.[7]

In recent years, the discovery that breast implants could cause cancer of the immune system (ALCL) supports the claim that breast implants can have a harmful impact on the immune system.

Treatments and Alternatives

Here are some symptoms that many women have reported to have developed after getting breast implants. Some of these symptoms developed almost immediately, but others developed years later.

- I have achy, sore, or weak muscles.
- I have achy or stiff joints.
- I wake up every morning feeling tired or un-refreshed, and no matter how much I sleep, I never feel well-rested.
- I feel like my head is in a "fog." I have difficulty concentrating, finding the right word to say, or remembering things.
- I feel warm or hot even when it's cold outside.
- I have dry skin, dry eyes, or hair loss.

If you already have an autoimmune disease, breast implants could make your symptoms worse. If autoimmune disease runs in your family, you may be at increased risk of developing an autoimmune reaction to the silicone implant. If you already have breast implants and have any of the above symptoms, here are some steps to consider:

- See a rheumatologist. A rheumatologist is a specialist of joint and immune system conditions. The rheumatologist can examine you and order tests if necessary to potentially diagnose any conditions. See a provider you trust and don't be afraid to get a second opinion. This is your right as a patient!
- Your doctor may offer you medications to treat your symptoms. For example, he/she may offer you artificial tears to

help with dry eyes or suggest medications to decrease inflammation in your body.

The Bottom Line

Although well-designed large, long-term studies are lacking, women with implants and autoimmune symptoms have reported for decades that their symptoms improved when their implants were removed. A Dutch study found that among 52 women who had their implants removed, 36 (69%) reported that they felt better, and 9 of the 36 reported that their symptoms were gone.[8] A meta-analysis, which is a type of study that combines the results from several studies, found that on average, 3 out of 4 women who removed their silicone breast implants saw improvement in their symptoms.[9]

However, the prognosis might be better for women with autoimmune symptoms who have their implants removed than for women with a diagnosed autoimmune disease.

All articles are reviewed and approved by Diana Zuckerman, PhD, and other senior staff.

1. U.S. FDA. Medical Devices: Breast Implants: Risks of Breast Implants. (Apr. 4, 2017). Available Online: https://www.fda.gov/MedicalDevices/ProductsandMedicalProcedures/ImplantsandProsthetics/BreastImplants/ucm064106.htm#Connective_Tissue_Disease.

2. Mentor. Mentor Silicone Gel-Filled Breast Implant Product Insert Data Sheet. (Nov. 2006). Available online: https://www.accessdata.fda.gov/cdrh_docs/pdf3/p030053c.pdf.

3. Cohen Tervaert JW, Colaris MJ, van der Hulst RR. Silicone breast implants and autoimmune rheumatic diseases: myth or reality. *Curr Opin Rheumatol.* 2017 Jul;29(4):348-354. doi: 10.1097/BOR.0000000000000391.

4. de Boer M, Colaris M, van der Hulst RRW, Cohen Tervaert JW.Is explantation of silicone breast implants useful in

patients with complaints? *Immunol Res.* 2017 Feb;65(1):25-36. doi: 10.1007/s12026-016-8813-y.

5. Maijers MC, et al. Women with silicone breast implants and unexplained systemic symptoms: a descriptive cohort study. The Netherlands Journal of Medicine. 2013; 71(10): 534-540. Available online: http://www.njmonline.nl/getpdf.php?id=1392. Brown SL, Pennello G, Berg WA, Soo MS, Middleton MS. "Silicone Gel Breast Implant Rupture, Extracapsular Silicone, and Health Status in a Population of Women." *The Journal of Rheumatology* 2001.

6. Brinton LA, Buckley LM, Dvorkina O et al. Risks of connective tissue disorders among breast implant patients. *American Journal of Epidemiology.* 2004; 180: 619-27.

7. Maijers MC, et al. Women with silicone breast implants and unexplained systemic symptoms: a descriptive cohort study. The Netherlands Journal of Medicine. 2013; 71(10): 534-540. Available online: http://www.njmonline.nl/getpdf.php?id=1392.

8. de Boer M, Colaris M, van der Hulst RRW, Cohen Tervaert JW.Is explantation of silicone breast implants useful in patients with complaints? *Immunol Res.* 2017 Feb;65(1):25-36. doi: 10.1007/s12026-016-8813-y.

National Center for Health Research
1001 Connecticut Avenue NW, Suite 1100
Washington, DC 20036

Are Your Implants Poisoning You?

Are Your Breast Implants Poisoning You?

Johane van den Berg, Longevity Magazine. June 18, 2018.

This information was taken directly from: http://www.center4research.org/breast-implants-poisoning/

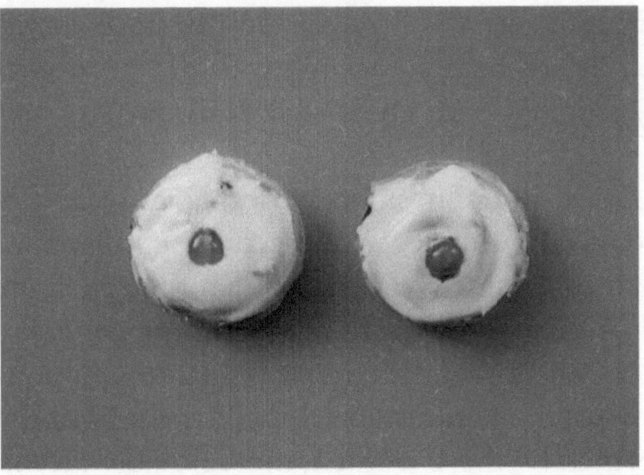

Victoria Beckham, Crystal Hefner, Pamela Anderson, Yolanda Hadid, Melissa Gilbert and Heather Morris. What do these famous women have in common with thousands of other women worldwide? Well, for one thing, they all decided to get breast implants when they were younger. And now all of them have decided to remove what many are referring to as their "toxic bags".

After their arrival on the cosmetic-surgery market in the 1960s, both silicone and saline breast implants quickly became the most popular plastic surgery procedure for women. According to the American Society of Plastic Surgeons, breast augmentation is still the number one surgical procedure for women, ranking above liposuction, nose reshaping, eyelid surgery and the tummy tuck. *The problem, explains Dr Diana Zuckerman, Ph.D. and President of the National Centre for Health Research in the United States, is that surgeons who administer breast implants often minimize the risks associated with this procedure.* Consequently, the majority of women don't realize that a few years after the procedure, they may need to have their implants removed. Additionally, they are unaware that removal costs at least as much as implantation.

This is despite the fact that various official organizations warn that breast implants should not be regarded as lifetime devices. The FDA in the US, for example, explains that the longer you have breast implants, the more likely it will be for you to have them removed. In addition, their list of risks associated with this procedure is extensive and detailed, ranging from chest wall deformity to toxic shock syndrome.

Now, about 50 years after breast implants were first introduced globally, un-tracked numbers of women are complaining of a recognizable pattern of health problems, which they attribute to their implants. Those suffering from these symptoms generally refer to the condition as Breast Implant Illness or BII (although non-medical, this term is widely used). Various social media groups and organizations have been formed by these women, most notably Healing Breast Implant Illness and The Implant Truth Survivors.

Symptoms of this condition — which Dr Zuckerman explains, is a pattern of health problems likely caused by an autoimmune reaction to the implant — include mental confusion, joint pain, hair loss, dry eyes, chronic fatigue, and persistent flu-like symptoms. "In some cases," she says, "silicone gel is leaking into their bodies and causing the autoimmune reaction. When the gel leaks into organs such as the lungs and liver, it can't be removed surgically."

In addition, a lot of women experience what is called capsular contracture. This occurs when the scar tissue around the implant (inside the body) gets tight and hard. This can make the breasts look abnormal and cause chronic pain and hardness.

But aren't breast implants supposed to be a safe procedure?

"In the context of health and longevity, it is urgent to dispel many current misconceptions about breast augmentation and other implant-based cosmetic surgery procedures," says Dr Pierre Blais. He is considered to be the world's foremost expert on breast implants as failed medical devices. He is also a former Canadian Government researcher and Senior Scientific Advisor. Dr Blais explains that, because implants are designed to be temporary devices, they degrade chemically and wear out, eventually releasing their content.

"The process is silent and insidious, as the released substances are aggressive and some are outright toxic or infective (for saline implants). Thus, with ageing, the implant site undergoes destructive anatomic and biochemical changes – termed necrosis – as tissue dies and solubilized proteins become denatured."

Moreover, in one of his papers on the topic, Dr Blais determines that implants can injure without undergoing mechanical failure. Studies on long-term implant users indicate that, in the pectoral and intercostal areas, gradual and irreversible deterioration of muscle function takes place. Respiratory problems are widespread among implant users, as are complications affecting major lymphatic ducts and fluid irrigation of the upper chest. Dr Blais has tested thousands of explanted tissue samples and capsules, finding that they are prone to not only various types of bacteria, but also yeast and mold.

How do implants contract these bacteria?

Although saline-filled implants are presented and regarded as the "safe" option compared to silicon – containing only salt and water – they are rarely hermetically 'sealed'. Moreover, their filling valves aren't perfectly secure. As a result, they allow the body fluids of the user to infiltrate, along with bacteria, yeast and molds. After this happens, decaying elements will start building up. When the shell eventually starts leaking into the user's chest, the contaminated contents is discharged and spread through the body.

Indeed, if given enough time, anyone who has breast implants will start to experience these symptoms. Dr Blais describes this as a form of local, accelerated biochemical ageing. Eventually the site of the implant will start to resemble a large chronic abscess, and secondary corrective surgery will be required in any case.

This is why, he explains, athletes and entertainment professionals who undergo breast augmentation, can expect a drastic decrease in stamina, appearance and comfort during their late career. This is known in medical and paramedical circles and explains why breast implants are sometime called "the time bandits".

According to an investigation involving a number of different patients done by CBS 5 – who also worked with Dr Blais to determine the validity of this condition – after explant, almost all of the autoimmune symptoms eventually disappear.

Are there any forms of breast implants that are considered safe?

"There are no breast implants on the market that never cause side effects or complications," says Dr Zuckerman. *"In general, breast implants filled with saline are less likely to cause serious injury than those filled with silicone gel, but we know many women who have become ill because of saline implants."*

Often, when a woman chooses to undergo this procedure, she is persuaded by her plastic surgeon (or breast surgeons after mastectomy) that breast implants are safe devices. Although there are thousands of stories of women whose health deteriorated as a result of their implants, the voice a plastic surgeon will more than often outweigh the information. This is because patients tend to hear what they want instead of making a decision based on information from both sides.

"Then, when women experience these complications," explains Dr Zuckerman, *"they are furious at themselves for making a decision based on limited information and furious at their doctors for not warning them of the risks. The women who are most harmed by breast implants are the ones that don't realize that their health is deteriorating because of their implants, or don't have $8,000-10,000 to get their implants removed by an experienced explant surgeon."*

C H A P T E R   3

Silicone Exposed

Here are some of the known toxic chemicals in silicone:

1. Methyl Ethyl Ketone
2. Cyclobexanone
3. Isopropyl Alcohol
4. Denatured Alcohol
5. Acetone
6. Urethane
7. Poly Vinyl Chloride
8. Lacquer Thinner
9. Ethyl Acetate
10. Epoxy Resin
11. Epoxy Hardener
12. Amine, Printing Ink
13. Toluene
14. Freon
15. Silica
16. Flux
17. Solder
18. Chlorplantinic Acid
19. Metal Cleaning Acid
20. Formaldehyde
21. Talcum Powder
22. Chlorplatinic Acid
23. Metal Cleaning Acid
24. Formaldehyde
25. Talcum Powder
26. Color Pigment Printers Ink
27. Oakite
28. Cyanoacyrylates
29. Ethylene Oxide
30. Carob Black
31. Xylene
32. Hexone
33. Benzene
34. Hexanone
35. Thixon-OSN-2
36. Rubber
37. Acid Stearic
38. Zinc Oxide
39. Naptha
40. Phenol
41. Methylene Chloride
42. Platinum Salts
43. Platinum
44. other heavy metals

I had allergen, non-textured implants. The outer shell was silicone, which was never mentioned to me at consult (pre-implant). The outer shell is just as toxic as the inside contents regardless of whether it is if filled with saline or silicone.

Detoxification of Silicone and Saline Breast Implants

This information was taken directly from: https://healingbreastimplantillness.com/detoxification/

Breast implants cause toxicity in the body several different ways. First, breast implants are large, foreign objects which engage the immune system on an ongoing basis eventually overwhelming the immune system and causing immune system dysfunction and failure. Immune system dysfunction leads to auto-immune symptoms and diseases. Immune system failure allows opportunistic organisms such as bacteria, fungi, viruses and parasites to grow unchecked and spread out of control. These bacteria, fungi, viruses and parasites produce bio-toxins which cause an inflammatory cascade and overload our organs of detoxification. Bacteria and fungus can cause or contribute to autoimmune diseases. Further, breast implants are essentially two large sacks of aggressive cyto-toxic, neuro-toxic and carcinogenic chemicals which are highly inflammatory to our tissues, organs and glands. Please see breast implant safety for a list of toxic chemicals in silicone implants. Inflammation and the body's natural systems of detoxification are body processes which work together like a teeter totter. When inflammation in the body increases due to breast implants, detoxification is down regulated by the body. When inflammation in the body decreases, detoxification is up regulated by the body. So, the presence of toxic implants in the body substantially increases inflammation which hampers the body's natural systems of detoxification. The entire time you have implants your systems of detoxification are diminished and you are collecting toxins from all sources. In addition, high inflammation from breast implants is known to cause disease and illness such as cancer, auto-immune diseases and metabolic diseases.

Further, silicone is a known adjuvant which causes auto-immune symptoms and diseases. Silicone chemicals are also known endocrine disruptors. Endocrine disruptors are chemicals that interfere with the bodies sensitive endocrine glandular system and produce adverse developmental, reproductive, neurological and immune effects. The endocrine glands especially hard hit by breast implants are thymus, thyroid and a doctrinal but this does not exclude the other glands such as pancreas, ovaries, parathyroid, pineal, pituitary and hypothalamus. Our glands essentially control all the processes in our body and damaging them with endocrine disruptors is very significant to our health.

Breast implants contain heavy metals. Over the years breast implant manufacturers have used different heavy metals in their silicone recipes. We are beginning to understand the causation that heavy metals plays in toxicity, illness and many of the diseases plaguing mankind. I phoned Mentor and asked what in the breast implants was making me so sick and they told me Platinum but they refused to divulge the other chemicals used in their manufacturing process of implants. It was not only Platinum that was making me ill, however Platinum is a known toxicity that they will admit to being in breast implants. Basically every chemical used to make silicone breast implants is toxic to our body.

CHAPTER 4

US to Investigate Health Impact of Nickel, Silicone in Medical Implants

This information was taken directly from: https://www.icij.org/investigations/implant-files/us-to-investigate-health-impact-of-nickel-silicone-in-medical-implants/

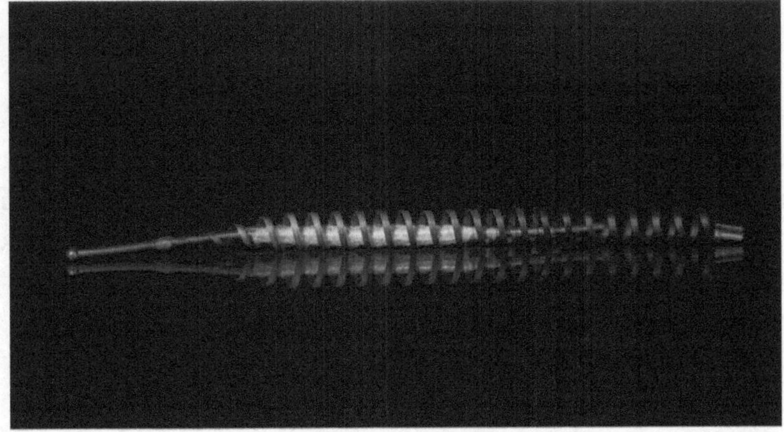

By Sasha Chavkin
March 18, 2019

A fresh U.S. Food and Drug Administration probe into adverse patient reactions to materials in medical devices, including breast implants, metal-on-metal hips and the birth control coil Essure, has been announced. The FDA says it will hold a public hearing this fall into nitinol as part of the investigation into inflammatory and immune responses in patients; it will task its own scientists to conduct research on medical implant materials; and it will review published studies. Nitinol is an alloy containing nickel that is used in Essure. Many patients have reported allergic reactions to Essure and the U.S. Centers for Disease Control have estimated that between 10 and 20 percent of the population is allergic to nickel.

The agency will also consider patient responses to the silicone contained in breast implants in a previously announced hearing on breast implant safety due to take place on March 25-26.
"We believe the current evidence, although limited, suggests some individuals may be predisposed to develop an immune/inflammatory reaction when exposed to select materials," the FDA said in its statement.
Last fall, the International Consortium of Investigative Journalists reported extensively on breast implants, Essure and metal-on-metal hips as part of the global Implant Files investigation of the medical device industry and its overseers. ICIJ's coverage examined regulators' refusal to recognize adverse reactions to these devices among patients, including breast implant illness, an ailment reported by many breast implant patients characterized by chronic fatigue, muscle pain and cognitive difficulties.

The announcement marks a shift in the agency's approach toward breast implant illness in just the last six months. On Sept. 14, 2018, after a study by the respected MD Anderson Cancer Center found elevated risks of autoimmune disease among patients with breast implants, the FDA issued a statement indicating that agency officials "respectfully disagree with the authors' conclusions." In its

March 15 announcement, the agency appeared more open to the possibility that breast implants could increase the risks of fatigue, muscle pain and cognitive issues among some patients.

"While the FDA doesn't have definitive evidence suggesting breast implants are associated with these conditions, we're looking to gain a fuller understanding of this issue to communicate risk, minimize harm and help in the treatment of affected patients," it stated.

The FDA is also increasing its scrutiny of nitinol. Last August, a law firm in Australia launched a class action lawsuit on behalf of patients alleging that their Essure implants corroded and caused them to suffer nickel poisoning. The suit is expected to be filed in May, said a spokeswoman for the law firm, Slater and Gordon.

Essure was withdrawn from the market worldwide at the end of 2018. However, the FDA noted that nitinol is used in other implants such as cardiovascular stents and guidewires, and said that it will issue draft guidelines in the coming months for the use of nitinol in medical devices.

Clarification, March 21, 2019: ICIJ has clarified this story to reflect that the Essure lawsuit in Australia was launched in August 2018 but has not yet been filed.

International Consortium of Investigative Journalists

1710 Rhode Island Ave NW, 11th floor, Washington DC 20036 USA
contact@icij.org

FDA Kept Hundreds of Thousands of Breast Implant Incidents Hidden From Public

This information was taken directly from: https://www.icij.org/investigations/implant-files/fda-kept-hundreds-of-thousands-of-breast-implant-incidents-hidden-from-public/

The U.S. Food and Drug Administration held a public hearing into breast implant safety.

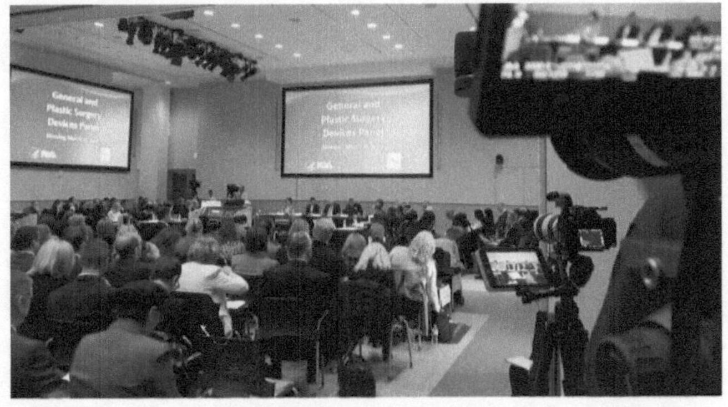

By Sasha Chavkin
March 25, 2019

On the eve of a hearing about the hidden dangers of breast implants, the U.S. regulator charged with informing the public about those risks revealed it has long known about vastly more injuries and other complications than it has previously disclosed. Since 2009, the U.S. Food and Drug Administration has received more than 350,000 incident reports involving breast implants, according to a chart shared by the agency. That's more than 20 times as many reports as the agency had posted on its public-facing database as of late last year.

As the International Consortium of Investigative Journalists reported in November, the FDA has allowed manufacturers to bury so-called adverse event reports using a program known as "alternative summary reporting." Once the FDA began requiring more complete disclosure, the number of injuries and other incidents surged, from a few hundred a year to more than 4,000 in 2017 and more than 8,000 in the first half of 2018.

But even those numbers are dwarfed by the agency's latest disclosure. About 90,000 reports came into the agency in those two years, according to the FDA. In recent years, the number of medical device reports (MDRs) submitted to the FDA in relation to breast implants have increased.

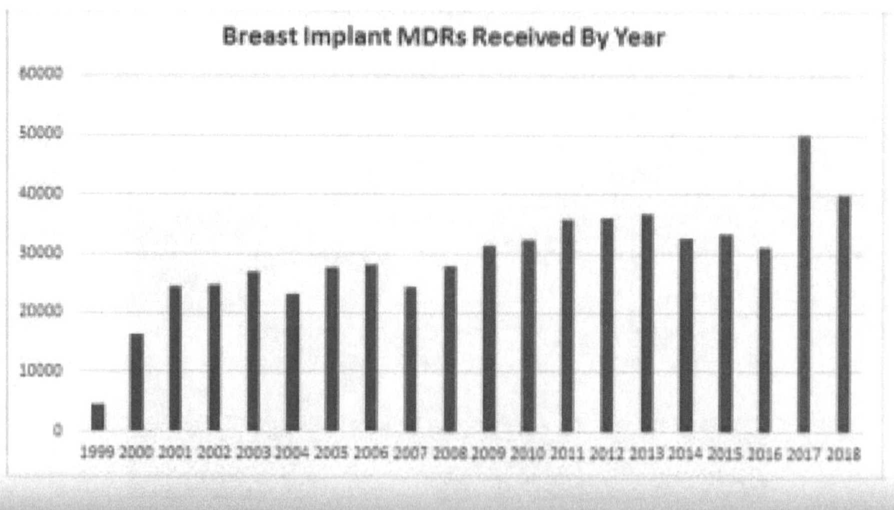

The statistics were disclosed in advance of an FDA hearing on breast implant safety that was dominated by women who said that they were not properly warned by their doctors and health authorities about the products' risks. "We have a much larger and more serious issue than we knew coming into this meeting," said Madris Tomes, a former FDA data analyst and the founder of Device Events, a database that tracks medical device adverse events data. "This means that we are dealing with an agency that is withholding the number of reports with no regard for the patients and physicians who seek to better understand the information."

The FDA did not provide a breakdown of the type of incidents described in the reports, making it unclear how many reflected serious injuries such as ruptures and infections and how many reflected product malfunctions that did not harm patients. FDA spokeswoman Stephanie Caccomo said the agency was reviewing the reports all along even though it was not disclosing them to the public.

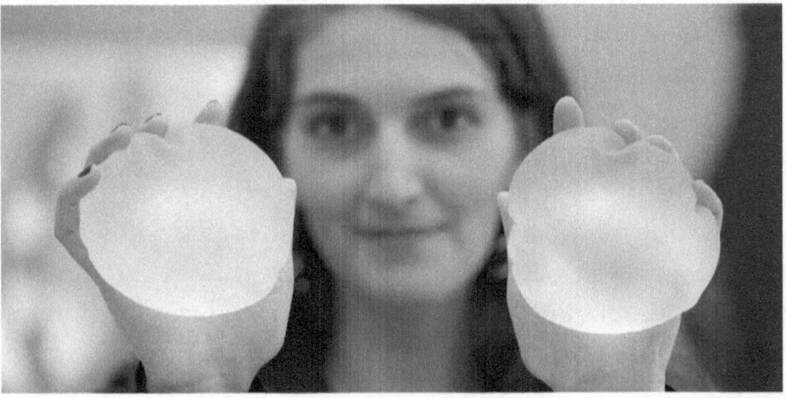

"The visibility of the reports does not change how the FDA was reviewing the reports," Caccomo said in response to ICIJ's inquiries about the new data. The table reflects the agency's "effort to promote greater public transparency," she said. More than 10 million women have received breast implants over the last decade. Most don't report any problems. But long-standing questions about durability have never been resolved. The FDA's own safety notices warn that as many as one in five women who receive breast implants will get them removed within a decade due to complications such as rupture, deflation and the painful contraction of scar tissue around the implant, known as capsular contracture.

Breast implants are also blamed by tens of thousands of patients, and a growing number of medical professionals, for a range of autoimmune-related ailments generally referred to as breast implant illness.

Dozens of patients who complain of breast implant-related health problems came to the FDA hearing, held at the agency's suburban campus in Silver Spring, MD. "Don't ignore us," testified Holly Davis of Charleston, South Carolina, who says she suffered severe memory loss, rashes and hair loss after getting breast implants. "We are real." Davis asked women in the audience who had gotten breast implants to stand, and asked them if they would get implants today if they had been properly warned of the potential hazards.
"No!" shouted back more than a dozen women in unison.

Patients regularly punctuated the proceeding with cheers and applause when experts and advocates spoke out against the products' risks. "Half our members are seeing breast implant illness patients," said Mindy Hawes, a plastic surgeon and member of the plastic surgeons' group Aesthetic Society. "We need to educate our members." Last week, the FDA announced an investigation into adverse patient reactions to silicone, marking a new openness to recognizing breast implant illness.

Another focus of the hearing, which will continue Tuesday, was a rare form of cancer called breast implant associated anaplastic large cell lymphoma (BIA-ALCL). BIA-ALCL is not a breast cancer, but a cancer of the immune system. Studies have shown that patients with a kind of implant known as a textured implant face a higher risk of BIA-ALCL. Textured implants produced by leading manufacturer Allergan were suspended from the European and Brazilian markets in December 2018 after losing their European certification. In February, a French government inquiry recommended that one brand of textured implants, Allergan Biocell, should be permanently banned.

In February, the FDA sent a letter to health providers across the U.S. warning them about the association between implants and BIA-ALCL. At the hearing, industry representatives detailed their research into BIA-ALCL and breast implant illnesses, and expressed sympathy for women have fallen ill. "We empathize with these women and can only imagine how distressing it is for them," said Stephanie Manson Brown, Vice President of Clinical Development for Allergan, on reports on breast implant illness.

Monday's panel did not take any votes or issue formal recommendations. The panel's deliberations will be used by the FDA in the following weeks and months as the agency considers whether to adopt additional restrictions or regulations on breast implants.

International Consortium of Investigative Journalists

1710 Rhode Island Ave NW, 11th floor
Washington DC 20036 USA
contact@icij.org

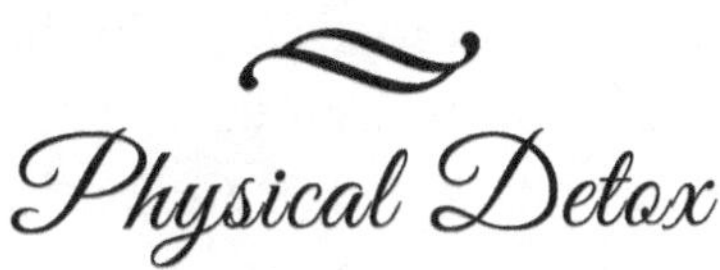

Physical Detox

This information was taken directly from: <u>https://healingbreastimplantillness.com</u>

STEPS TO DETOXIFY YOUR BODY FROM SILICONE AND SALINE BREAST IMPLANTS

1. Explant – The first and most important step to detox the body is to properly explant your breast implants which means En Bloc/Total Capsulectomy. Please see the **explant** page for a full explanation of a proper explant and the **explant surgeons** page for a list of worldwide surgeons who remove breast implants properly. After explant give your body a month to recover and heal from surgery before stimulating detoxification.

2. Diet – The next and most important step after removal of breast implants is to support the body's natural systems of detoxification through healthy diet which means an organic, nonGMO, whole foods diet of little fruit, (lemons, limes, coconut, green granny smith apples and berries are the best fruits to eat) lots and lots of all kinds of vegetables (50 per cent raw 50 per cent cooked), some organic/

free range/grass fed meats and eggs, some resistant starch carbs to feed probiotics and some carbs from root vegetables. Include lots of healthy fats and oils such as organic/raw/grass fed butter if you can tolerate dairy, coconut oil, unheated olive oil, avocado and avocado oil, fresh flax seed oil and lots of clean fish/krill oils. Include raw nuts except peanuts which carry mold. Drink six to eight glasses of purified, mineralized water. Cut out all sugars/sweeteners, dairy and gluten which are inflammatory to most guts. Cut out all processed foods, anything with a label on it, anything in a can, anything in a box, cut out all chemicals, cut out all sweets, candies, cakes, pastries, cut out caffeine, pop, chocolate, alcohol, yeasted and foods with vinegar. Use a natural sea or celtic salt full of various minerals from a clean source. Use apple cider vinegar.

Your clean, wholefoods diet will be the most important factor in how you feel day to day and how quickly your body detoxes. Eating cleanly allows your body the extra energy it needs to do the heavy work of detoxing. Examples of diets that work for us are the Gerson Therapy diet (good for vegetarians), antifungal/low mycotoxin diets (good for fungus which many of us battle for months after explant) and the AutoImmune Protocol diet (good for those that suffer from autoimmune symptoms and diseases). These diets are digestible to the body, lower inflammation in the gut and do not feed fungus and other pathogenic microorganisms that cause many of our symptoms.

3. Heal Your Gut – Many women who have toxicity from breast implants have digestion and bowel problems potentially from leaky gut, gut dysbiosis, IBS, Crohns, inflammation, fungus and parasites. Some women develop allergies due to leaky gut and lose the ability to digest dairy, gluten grains, and other inflammatory or allergenic foods. All inflammatory and allergic foods must be cut out of the diet completely in order to lower inflammation in the gut and support digestion. When inflammation is present in the gut and digestive tract the body slows down or stops digestion and detoxification. If you have gut problems, a whole foods diet as outlined above and cutting out inflammatory and allergenic foods such as dairy and gluten will help you feel better, digest better and detox faster. Bone broth and powdered collagen will help heal your gut and please ensure you have enough Betaine HCL to digest your food. If your gut is badly damaged and not responding to good diet and bone broth and you need additional help please check out the GAPS diet guidelines for healing damaged guts. If you have auto-immune symptoms follow the Autoimmune Protocol diet to bring down inflammation in your gut and modulate the autoimmune response in the body.

Probiotics, especially lactic acid producing and soil based probiotics found in fermented foods such as yogurt and cultured vegetables and raw vegetables are very important for healing/restoring healthy gut flora and function, modulating your immune system and chelating toxins from the body. If you buy sauerkraut, obtain it from a health food store which carries traditionally cultured veggies and avoid grocery store ones made with vinegar. It is easy and inexpensive to make your own cultured vegetables at home which supply much larger quantities of probiotics than store bought supplements. Just google Doctor. Mercola Cultured Vegetables Recipe and you will find a link to a great video on how to make your own cultured veggies if you are inclined. If you prefer to buy probiotics look for lactic acid based which means they produce lactic acid and look for soil based probiotics and take several doses each day for a long while to bring your gut flora, digestion and bowels back to normal. Rotate your probiotics to get a good cross section of various organisms.

4. Check for MTHFR Gentic Variants and Support your Methylation and Detox Pathways – MTHFR genetic variants which are easy to treat if present may be inhibiting your ability to detox if left untreated. In polls taken in our Facebook group more than half of the respondents had MTHFR genetic variants which inhibit our methylation and detoxing. Many test for MTHFR through their doctor or through 23andme.com. MTHFR is easy to treat with a few supplements such as methylfolate, methylB12 and MethylB6 or Hy-doctoroxyB12. My MTHFR status accounted for some of my own particular illness picture including my level of toxicity from breast implants and heavy metals and my very low B12 status which caused many of my symptoms. Many women in the group have low B12 due to years with breast implants and toxicity from breast implants. B12 is crucial to many processes in our body and crucial to our detoxing.

5. Infections In Us – After explant, some ladies have discovered fungal colonization in their saline implants and chest. Some ladies have had contact with mold in their environment and have mold infections in their body due to immune deficits caused by breast implants. Additionally, most breast implant illness ladies have an overgrowth of fungus such as yeast/Candida in their gut and even systemically in their body due to immune deficits. Many ladies also have other infections in their gut such as H-pylori and SIBO. Some ladies had bacterial infections in their capsules. Capsular contracture is known to be caused by bacteria in the capsule. Some ladies have mycoplasma infections. Some ladies have Lyme, EBV and herpes infections causing their health problems. These bacterial, mold/fungus, mycobacteria, viral and parasitical infections caused by immune deficits due to breast implants need to be eliminated for a full recovery. Sometimes these infections can be detected through various tests but not always. Bacterial infections are treated with antibiotics. Mold should be treated with mold eliminating protocols by doctors knowledgeable about mold such as Functional Medicine doctors knowledgeable about Doctor. Ritchie Shoemaker's Protocol. Gut and broad fungal infections in most of us such as yeast/Candida are treated with antifungal/low mycotoxin diets and antifungals whether natural or prescription. Antifungal/low mycotoxin diets are crucial to overcoming mold and fungus in the body and strict diet supersedes prescription antifungals. Fungus/mold overcomes prescription antifungals quickly. Treating with too many prescription antifungals is causing resistant fungus and prescription antifungals can be hard on the liver. Use natural antimicrobials if possible. A glass of hot water with the juice of one lemon and cayenne pepper first thing every morning cleans out the digestive tract daily. Three cloves of crushed garlic a day, one with each meal kills fungus while preserving beneficial gut flora. Oil of Oregano drops several times a day also kills fungus. Grapefruit Seed extract kills fungus. A product called Thorne Research SF722 is excellent for killing fungus, Caprylic Acid/Caprylates and Candex kills yeast/Candida powerfully. There are many good natural products to eliminate fungus in your body. Rotate your natural antifungals every month or sooner so the fungus does not build up a tolerance to them.

6. Support your Endocrine and Immune System – Consider checking your Cortisol levels with a pm Cortisol blood test or a Four Point Cortisol test and check your thyroid's free T3, T4 conversion to see if your adrenals and thyroid are functioning properly. You may need to support both adrenals and thyroid in order to get well. There are various supplements that will help support your endocrine and immune system. Echinacea, Epicor, Tansfer Factors Multi Immune are known as good supplements to support the immune system as are certain mushrooms such as Reishi. Vitamin C and zinc support the immune system too.

7. Progesterone – Progesterone stimulates your natural, nightly detoxification cycle and helps balance your hormones. As silicone is an endocrine disruptor and estrogenic in nature (acts like estrogen in the body) and toxic chemicals and heavy metals damage thyroid, adrenals and ovaries, some ladies have hormonal imbalances and are low on progesterone and other hormones. Have your hormone levels tested and supplement with bio-identical hormones and especially progesterone if you are low so that you feel better, heal better and your natural cycle of detoxification is working. If you have to supplement estrogen avoid oral medications because they slow your liver detoxification cycle down and cause fungus to proliferate in the gut. I had to take bio-identical but as I healed I was able to wean off of them.

8. Green Vegetable Juicing – Vegetable juicing is very helpful to supply extra nutrition, potassium and enzymes crucial for healing and detoxification. Try and include a large vegetable juice in your diet each day. I found the Gerson Therapy Green Juice here very helpful to how I felt day to day and to my overall healing:
http://gerson.org/pdfs/Green_Juice_Recipe_and_Preparation.pdf

9. Remineralization – Minerals are required for every aspect of your body and for detoxification. I suggest putting a pinch of high quality celtic or sea salt and a couple drops of ionic liquid minerals in each glass of water to get various minerals on an ongoing basis. Most of us are so low on magnesium that it is drastically affecting our health. Magnesium is important to cell and muscle function and how you feel day to day and is usually very low in toxic and stressed people. Magnesium malate or magnesium glycinate is the preferable source for magnesium. Calcium may be required, too, especially if you cannot eat dairy foods. Toxic chemicals in the implants are very acidic as are biotoxins and the body leaches calcium from bones and teeth in an attempt to offset the acidity which causes sharp bone pain and tooth degradation. Use plant derived calcium which is more easily absorbed by your body. Potassium is a very important mineral to cells for healing and detoxification. If you are eating plenty of fruits and veggies and doing some green juicing each day you should be getting enough potassium. Use ionic liquid mineral supplements to replace the more trace minerals. Get a Hair Test to test yourself for low minerals and elements that may need shoring up so you can heal.

10. Vitamins and Antioxidant Supplements to Lower Inflammation and Support Healing – Vitamin and antioxidant supplements help keep inflammation low which stimulates detoxification. Please carefully read all labels and research supplements that you take as some have unhealthy ingredients. Vitamins A, B, C, E, Selenium, Zinc, CoQ10, Turmeric, Ginger and Krill will help lower inflammation in your body and keep your detoxification cycle up regulated. Vitamin D is important to healing and is the vitamin that controls hormones and is low in most of us. Most of us are very low in B vitamins and especially B12. Many find Meyer's Cocktail Vitamin IV's very helpful in their healing. Acetylcholine can be a major supplement in our healing too as it stimulate the Vagus nerve to lower inflammation and eliminates brain fog. Acetylcholine can be found in lecithin supplements.

11. Stimulate Detox – After you have mastered good diet and your digestion and bowels are working well, you may want to begin to stimulate detoxification. There are certain supplements that stimulate and speed up detoxification such as Vitamin C, Magnesium, Chlorella/Spirulina, Lipoic Acid, MSM, Inositol (for silicone detoxification), NAC (N-Acetyl L-Cysteine) and Iodine. Do your research on these and go slow. Try one at a time, taking smaller doses to begin with to test for tolerance and gradually titrating up your doses to stimulate detoxification until you feel symptoms. Then rest for some days while those toxins clear and then repeat. Don't take Chlorella, Lipoic Acid or NAC if you have mercury fillings as it will drag mercury around your body which is very toxic and causes inflammation. When you stimulate detoxification strongly, try a binder to bind toxins and help carry them out of the body. I like Chia seeds in a smoothie or water for a good daily binder. Start with 1 tsp of Chia seeds in 8 ounces of liquid and work up to 1 TBSP. If you need a stronger binder you can use charcoal but take care and do not use it for periods of longer than three weeks as charcoal binds healthy minerals and nutrients too.

12. Glutathione – If you do research on detoxification you will come across information on Glutathione which is a simple molecule produced in the body that acts as the body's master detoxifier picking up free radicals, toxins and heavy metals and escorting them out of the body. Normally, Glutathione is created and recycled in the healthy body except when the toxic load becomes too great and then it becomes depleted. Glutathione is made from the amino acids (protein building blocks) Cysteine, Glutamine and Glycine. If you want to increase your Glutathione you can take the inexpensive supplements NAC (N-Acetyl L-Cysteine) 4 parts, Glutamine 2 parts and Glycine 1 part in a glass of water between meals. No need to buy expensive Glutathione supplements. Alternatively, you can also take organic, grass fed, undenatured whey powder which has all the precursors to make Glutathione. Again, start slow taking one dose of NAC/Glutamine/Glycine in the beginning and working your way up.

13. Exercise – Get exercise each day if possible. At first walking, yoga and swimming are great exercises for healing breast implant illness. Gradually work up to fast walking and even jogging to get your circulation and lymph moving well. Go outside for fresh air and sun and to connect with nature each day. If possible, sit or lie on the ground/grass/beach each day to eliminate inflammation in your body through grounding.

14. Sauna Therapy and Epsom Salt Baths – If you have access to an infrared sauna, sauna two to three times each week. It is well known that toxins and heavy metals are eliminated through the skin by sweating and infrared kills microbes in the body. Avoid saunas if you have implants and or mercury fillings. Also take a couple Epsom salt baths a week for magnesium replenishing and detoxification.

15. Low Level Light Therapy, Oxygen Therapy, Ozone Therapy – I read another lady's site that said she had profound healing after receiving low level light therapy treatments on her chest to break down capsule tissue which should have been removed but was not. Not only did the low level light therapy breakdown the capsule tissue, it also killed the bacteria and fungus in her chest. Although I have not had a chance to try it, I believe it works and could be a profound healing tool for some. Chiropractors use low level light therapy in their practices, hopefully you can find one near you. I have personally tried oxygen therapy and it does stimulate healing. Many are having good results getting rid of bacteria, mold/fungus and viruses using ozone.

16. Timeframe to Feel Healthy – You will notice that the process of detoxification does increase inflammation in the body and the feeling of illness for a period. Moving toxic chemicals, bio-toxins and heavy metals through your body and organs will cause inflammation and detox symptoms (headaches, brain fog, negative mentalism, emotionalism, sore back bone, sore joints, general illness, fatigue, digestive disturbances) and an increase of your specific symptoms which is why you should go slow and need to take rests from detoxing but always maintain your clean wholefoods diet and some exercise if possible. Detoxification of breast implants is not a straight line, but rather an up and down process generally lasting one to two years. After explant, you will notice certain symptoms go away and you will feel better for a few months but then in a few months after explant, your body will begin the heavy work of detoxing stored chemicals and heavy metals from your cells and your symptoms will increase and go up and down for some months but gradually disappear one by one. Most women feel substantially better within about one or two years. If you are not improving over months and years, then you need to look for other sources of toxicity. Perhaps you have a bacterial or fungal infection that is creating bio-toxins. Please ensure you are not living or working in a moldy environment. Perhaps you have mercury toxicity from your amalgams or a dental event. Perhaps you have root canals that are producing potent bacteria creating illness in your body. Perhaps you have parasites. Keep looking for toxicity and keep working on elimination and detoxification.

Most of the above are things I did to get well. I was able to research a lot on the processes of detoxification and I tried a lot of things. I hurt myself sometimes by speeding up detox too much and unleashing more heavy metals and toxins than my body and organs were able to handle at one time. So, take care. If you try the supplements, add one thing at a time so you can tell if something bothers you. Not everyone will be able to tolerate all of these things and especially in the beginning of your healing. If you have a bad reaction, stop everything and rest. Then add one thing back in at a time so you can tell what is causing the reaction. Trust your own instincts. Personally, I did not get help from the medical doctors. Medical doctors don't believe that silicone is toxic and do not have training in diagnosing heavy metals poisoning or detoxification. One Naturopath told me that mercury fillings are okay and not to disturb them. Ridiculous! There is only one other substance on earth more toxic than mercury which is radioactive Plutonium. I often get asked if I am fully recovered. My explant was Jan 2013 and in the five years since my explant I have regained about 95 per cent of my health. Two years post explant I was approximately 65 to 70 per cent recovered. I was still healing in my third year. In the fourth year of my healing I discovered I had very low B12 and HydoctoroxyB12 shots healed the rest of my symptoms. It takes time to heal this illness and the damage we have done to our bodies so be patient with yourself and trust in your healing.

C H A P T E R   7

FDA Slams Breast Implant Makers

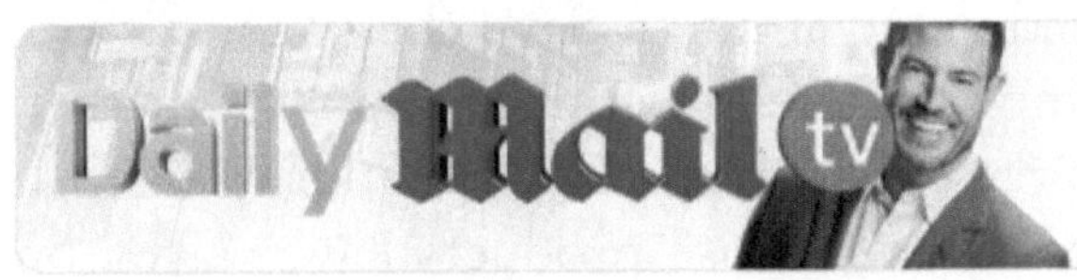

This information was taken directly from:

https://www.dailymail.co.uk/health/article-6830583/FDA-is-sues-warning-letters-breast-implant-manufacturers-days-hearing.html?ito=facebook_share_fbia-top&fbclid=IwAR0rAmh-k6NZDDDiLdXllcTEoTGgiMm9JFxJ8aB3bvCB3PpT7CXSvmFZ-9kzM

FDA slams breast implant makers in warning letters days before federal hearing that could BAN them from the US market

- **The US FDA slammed Mentor and Sientra for historically failing to complete the safety studies required for medical devices to stay on the market**
- **Breast implants are graded class III medical devices, requiring lengthy human studies to prove their safety**

- **The FDA warned the makers their products could be pulled if they don't provide more thorough data within 15 days**
- **Earlier this year, the FDA published data showing 9 women have died of and 457 have been diagnosed with BIA-ALCL, a rare cancer related to breast implants**

Days before a hearing on breast implant safety, US regulators have sent warning letters to two of the top implant manufacturers involved. In the letters, the US Food and Drug Administration reprimanded Mentor and Sientra for historically failing to complete the safety studies required for medical devices to stay on the market. f the firms do not have completed data within 15 days, the FDA warned, their blockbuster silicone implants could be pulled from the market. The warning is a gesture to patients that the FDA intends to be firm with breast implant manufacturers, whose products have stayed on the market for years without adequate safety data, despite ranking in the highest-risk bracket for medical devices. It comes amid global concerns over the safety of silicone breast implants, which have been officially linked to cancer of the immune system, and are alleged to cause autoimmune disorders.

Dr Diana Zuckerman, president of the National Center for Health Research, said the letters were 'surprising but encouraging' for US patients. 'I was surprised, but this is not the first time that the FDA has sent warning letters to implant companies that they are not complying with their research requirements,' Dr Zuckerman, a scientist who studies patient data and health after years in Congress overseeing committees on medical devices, told DailyMail.com. 'The important question is what the impact of those letters will be. Will the letters scare the companies enough that they improve their research? If not, will the FDA rescind approval of their products? The FDA has never rescinded approval of a device in those circumstances, and as long as FDA doesn't follow through on their threats, the companies don't have an incentive to improve their research. And if the research isn't improved, patients will still lack the information they need to make informed medical decisions.'

The US banned silicone implants in 1992, after 10 years of pushing industry for safety data to no avail. But companies immediately mounted plans to get the incredibly lucrative product back into the most lucrative market. Conferring with the FDA, they were able to keep administering the products to women in the US for the purpose of research. The firms presented their data in 2004, but the FDA rejected their application as poor in quality. Seventy-five percent of women dropped out of the Mentor trial before their first follow-up. In 2006, firms submitted three years of data - far less than the 10 years required - and the FDA conceded, on the grounds that companies engage in rigorous 10-year studies including at least 40,000 women.

Specifically, the FDA wanted to know the risks of rupture, leaks, scars contracting, difficulties performing mammograms around implants, links to lupus, and links to cancer. To this date, nobody has seen complete data from those studies the firms promised to complete. Until 2011, these gaps in data were dismissed as a work in progress. But then the FDA, alongside regulators around the world, published a statement saying there is strong evidence silicone breast implants are linked to BIA-ALCL, a rare cancer of the immune system. Since, thousands of women have reported autoimmune reactions, ruptures, scars contracting, and cancer. Earlier this year, the FDA published data showing nine women have died and 457 have contracted BIA-ALCL related to breast implants.

The hearing on Monday and Tuesday is a bid to interrogate all of the major players in the market, amid pressure from researchers, patient groups, and other regulators around the world (France, for example, has banned Allergan's silicone implants).The letters sent out to Mentor and Sientra focused on two products in particular. The Mentor implant is called MemoryShape, approved in 2013. On approval, Mentor agreed to conduct a specifically designed post-approval study. The FDA cites 'several serious deficiencies in the manufacturer's post-approval study', including low numbers of patients involved, a poor follow-up rate, and data inconsistencies, particularly failure to account for racial and ethnic disparities. Sientra's Silicone Gel Implants, also approved in 2013 with an order to study them after, followed a similar fate.

The FDA slammed the poor follow-up rate of just 61 percent, and accused Sientra of doing little to improve that. Mentor, which was reprimanded for having a history of inadequate data, slammed the warning letter, insisting the firm has tried to work with the FDA to get the right data. 'Mentor is disappointed with the FDA's decision to issue a Warning Letter despite our good faith efforts to address post-approval study requirements and without informing Mentor previously about any significant deficiencies,' the company said in a statement. 'In addition, a number of the details cited in the Warning Letter are incorrect and incomplete and we look forward to the opportunity to further discuss these discrepancies and next steps with the FDA.'

Sientra has yet to respond to DailyMail.com's request for a comment.

Idaho Mom Issues Breast Implant Warning

This information was taken directly from:

www.eastidahonews.com/2019/02/local-mom-issues-warning-after-breast-implant-nightmare/?fbclid=IwAR0CL-k87PGalzcnOni-wx7Hx4-EkJQWaw_rx5r_enRRbt8bGyQzL6e1V5hM

Natalia Hepworth, EastIdahoNews.com

Published at 7:40 pm, February 4, 2019

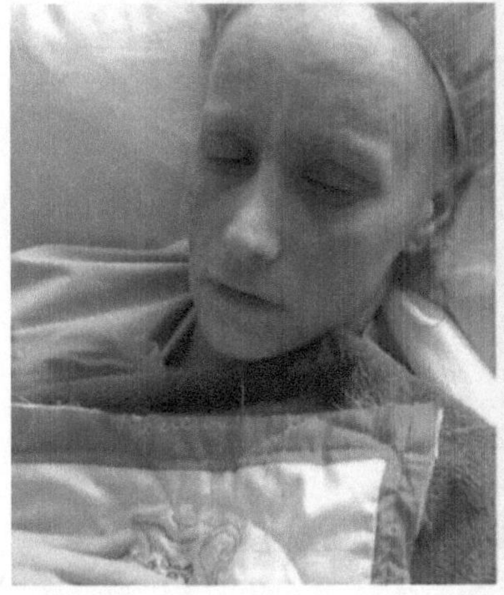
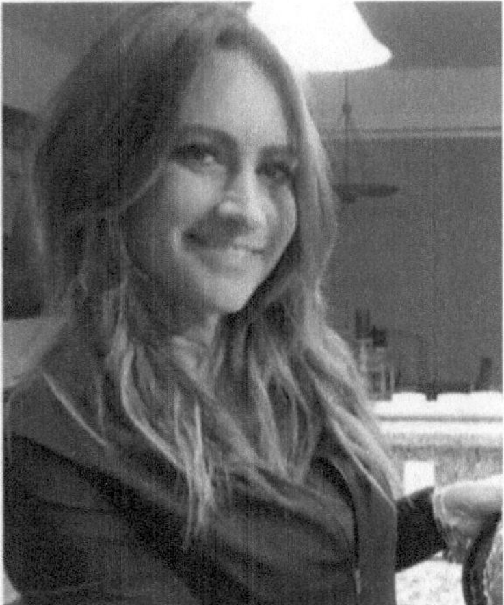

IDAHO FALLS — For Liza Hanks, the phrase "mom bod" accurately described her self-image after having two kids. "I felt like having children had taken a lot of that perkiness, and I felt like, 'I want to get breast implants,'" she says. Hanks was highly unsatisfied with the look of her breasts, and she thought implants were a lasting solution.

The decision

In 2008 Hanks underwent breast augmentation. Plastic surgeons inserted saline implants, and Hanks felt a new found confidence. Years passed without an issue, and Hanks enjoyed the look of her implants. But in 2015, her health began to take a turn for the worse, and she soon found the implants weren't worth the risk. "I found a lump in my right breast, and I went in for a mammogram scared to death that it was breast cancer," Hanks recalls. During a mammogram, a patient's breast is placed on a flat support plate and compressed with a parallel plate called a paddle. Hanks says the pressure of the machine pushed the implant in her right breast down, and she heard a tear as the right saline implant "bottomed out." "I was lopsided, but more importantly they found a golfball-sized mass in my right side. They said, 'You have to get this out, and it has to be biopsied for cancer,'" Hanks says.

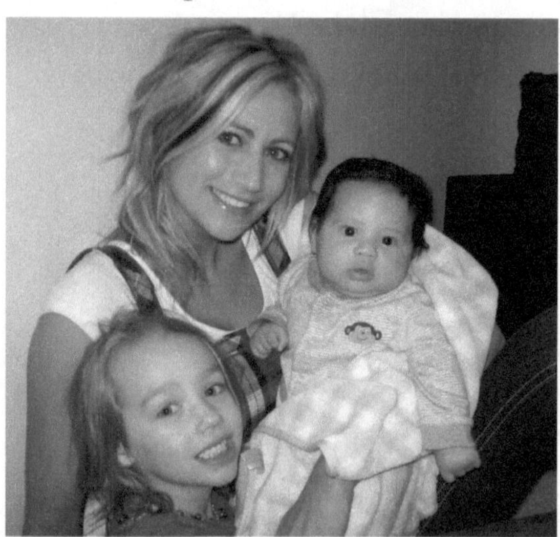

Liza Hanks before getting her first set of breast implants. | Courtesy photo

She set the critical appointment to have the mass removed, as well as a replacement for her implants. "I thought, 'Well, it's time to upgrade. It's time to get a new set in,'" Hanks says. Many women with implants have them replaced every seven to 10 years, so Hanks dropped $10,000 on new textured 'gummy bear' silicone implants that were expected to have a longer life than her old saline ones. Doctors removed the lump, which was benign. But when Hanks awoke from her procedure, she didn't feel quite like herself. "I knew immediately something was wrong," Hanks says.

Breast implant illness

Over the weeks and months following the surgery, Hanks experienced a myriad of symptoms and more than just an allergic reaction to the 40-plus chemicals found in a breast implant. It first started with the discoloration around her eyes. "They were just purple and red. They would burn, and it was really hard to see out of them. I went to various doctors to try and figure out what was causing this weird reaction," Hanks says. In conjunction with those symptoms, Hanks' incisions weren't healing. She experienced inflammation, confusion, extreme levels of anxiety, muscle aches and food intolerances. Soon her skin started shedding, her hair was falling out, and she dramatically lost weight.

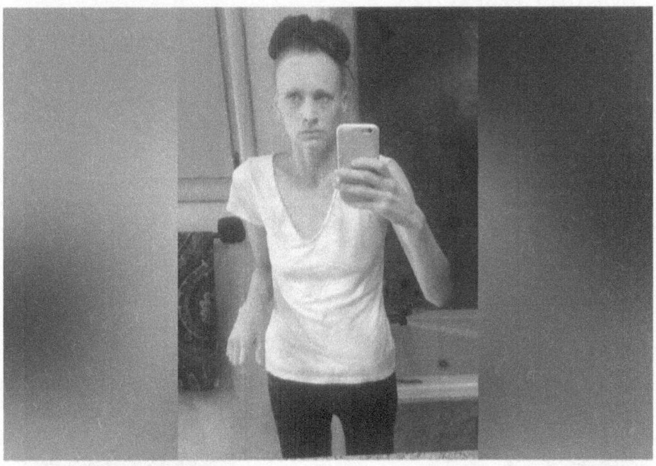

Doctors say Liza Hanks had an autoimmune inflammatory response to her textured silicone 'gummy bear' breast implants | Courtesy photos

"Common sense says, 'It's the implants. You just got implants,' but there were so many studies done by the implant manufacturers that it couldn't be the implants,' especially where breast implant illness is not recognized by the majority of the medical community," Hanks says. Hanks says she was dying, and her 31-year-old body began to take the shape of a 92-year-olds.

Her last chance

While weighing 87 pounds, Hanks' parents brought her to see Dr. Jeffrey Baker, an old friend who was practicing medicine in Idaho Falls. "When Liza came to me, she was really sick," Baker recalls. "I'm good friends with her dad, and he basically said, 'We need someone to help save Liza. She's so sick.'" Baker is an obstetrician/gynecologist who runs the Healing Sanctuary. Over the last decade, he's become familiar and certified in integrative functional medicine. He says Hanks was a medical mystery when she came to see him, and she was "really sick."

It took some time to get to the root cause of Hanks' issue, and he thought the implants might have been the root of the problems. He's had patients similar to Hanks, but the symptoms weren't nearly as potent. He tried various medical methods to try to restore Hanks' health, but nothing worked.

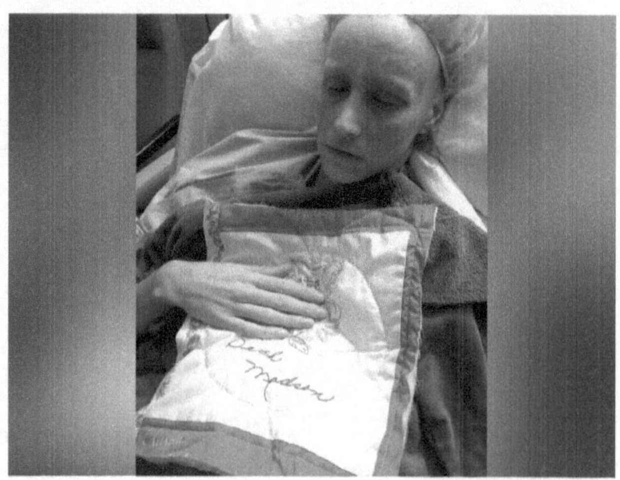

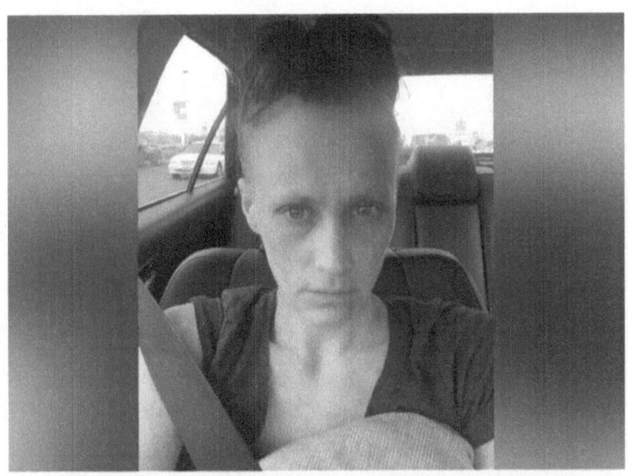

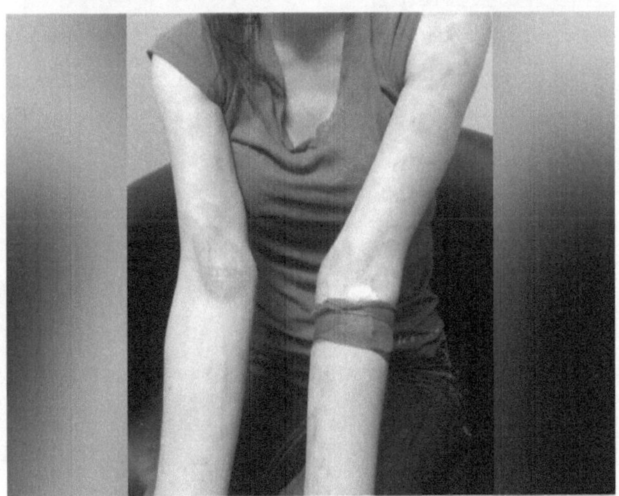

Liza Hanks says she was dying and because of her implants.
She was constantly experiencing a burning sensation. | Courtesy photos

"You could see her body trying to get rid of whatever was damaging it," Baker says. One day Baker came to a decision. He told Hanks she needed to have the implants removed. "The whole story and the whole journey points down to those implants. I told her, 'I really think you need to get those out,' because we couldn't find any other real source," Baker says.

Removing the implants

Hanks accepted the answer as her last chance at life and went back to the plastic surgeon who placed the implants. "(I said), 'Look I don't have much time, but I want the implants out. I do believe that this is the answer,'" Hanks says. "He said, 'You're just too sick. You're too ill, and I really don't want to do the surgery. I don't think you're healthy enough.'" Hanks persisted, and with Baker's help, the implants were removed the next day. "I remember waking up. … I took my first full breath and I no longer felt like I was burning alive on the inside," Hanks says. From there, her progress was immediate. Her vision, skin and hair follicles began healing. "I walked in two weeks after post-op into my plastic surgeon. I bounced in there, and I was like, 'Hey I'm alive,' and he was like, 'Wow,'" Hanks says.

Suffering leads to purpose

Hanks says she was lucky and blessed to find the right specialist to help her, and she's taken on her second chance at life in finding a positive purpose behind her suffering. "I was very, very lucky and blessed to find the right specialist that could say. 'Hey, you definitely had an autoimmune inflammatory response to breast implants and silicone, and thank goodness you got them out,'" Hanks says.

In 2017, more than 300,000 women and teenagers underwent surgery to have their breasts enlarged with silicone or saline implants, according to National Center for Health Research. The majority of surgeries result in little or no complications, but Hanks wants to help those who suffer following their procedures.

"There are a lot of women in the (online) breast implant illness groups that talk about how they can not find one doctor to back them and to support breast implant illness. I found four. I had incredible, amazing (doctors) — one of which I ended up marrying," Hanks says.

After Hanks' explant surgery, she dated ENT surgeon Dr. Kevin Hanks, who was instrumental in her recovery. Although she wasn't his patient, he was able to find the right team of medical professionals who could further aid in her recovery. Through his support and other local physicians, Hanks was able to get back on the road to healing.

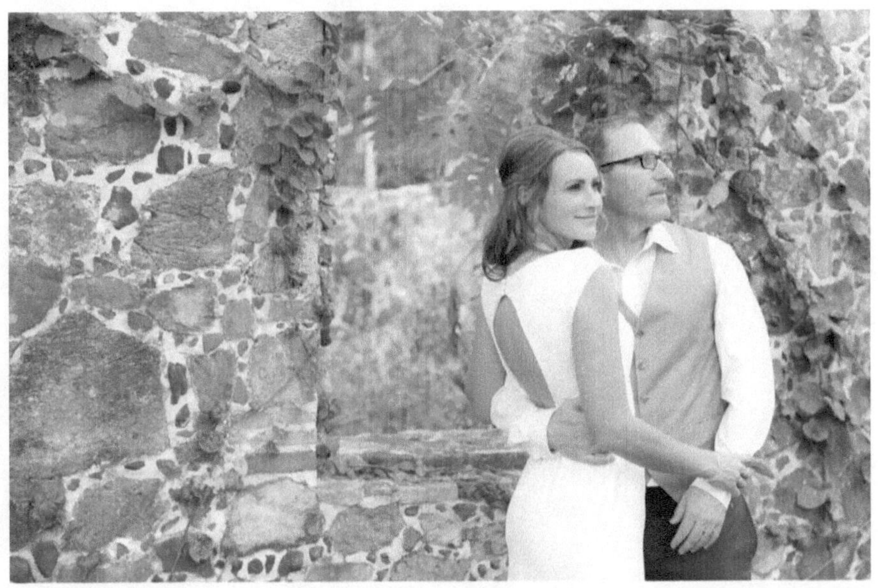

Liza Hanks and her husband Dr. Kevin Hanks. | Courtesy Photo

She now feels it's her responsibility to advocate for women and raise awareness about breast implant illness and those thinking of getting implants. "They're not totally safe. The 40-plus ingredients that make up a breast implant are not infallible in your body. They can rupture, they can leak, they can seep into your body," Hanks says. "There is limited research about breast implants. I feel like women deserve more information out there."

Hanks has joined other social media advocates and shares her health updates and story on her personal Instagram page. She's also working on writing a book about her breast implant illness journey. "I still see people that saw me on my deathbed and (they're) completely blown away," Hanks says. "That's why I'm an advocate for breast implant illness."

SECTION III

The Have's and the Have Not's

C H A P T E R   1

To Women with and Without Implants

Women with Implants:

To all the women out there who have implants, be encouraged. There is hope. There is help. I understand the financial strain of explanting but it must be done. If you are experiencing any of the symptoms previously mentioned it is well worth your time and money to investigate. Find a good doctor who understands the illness which accompanies breast implants. Serious if not fatal results are common with implants and they must not go unchecked.

I fully understand the intensity of the problems associated with implants. Autoimmune issues have a wide range of symptoms and they are as real as cancer or other health issues. You are not crazy. You are not a hypochondriac. You aren't making up symptoms so as to get of obligations or garner attention. You are sane and of sound mind. Your body is not lying to you. Something is wrong, very wrong and it can be fixed. I encourage you to visit the Facebook page:

https://healingbreastimplantillness.com

There you will read posts from thousands of women across the globe dealing with the same issues as you. They offer help, tell their stories, share their trials, and offer advice and the names of excellent

85

doctors who can and will aid in this matter. You are not alone and you do not have to go through this by yourself. I promise from personal experience that all these matters can come to a close with explanting.

Women Considering Implants:

My best advice: DON'T DO IT! If you can avoid it altogether, please do. The fewer foreign substances you put in your body the better. I fully understand that your reasons for getting them can range from low self-worth, feeling you will attract more men, you will feel better about yourself, mastectomy from cancer, trying to hang on to a cheating man who likes big breasts, you name it. I know there are varying reasons but none are worth jeopardizing your health. Most of the women who testify about BII say the implants did not boost their self-esteem nor did it make them feel better, prettier, sexier; at least not like they thought they would. Of course, that isn't all women, but you see my point.

Ladies, if you are thinking about getting them for superficial reasons, there are far better and safer ways to feel better about yourself. No man is worth harming your body. No man is worth the physical pain I have endured. If he is worth keeping, he will love, value and appreciate you just as you are. A real man does not place value on the size or shape of your breasts.

In the next chapter I will talk about the spiritual aspect of healing because, ultimately, there is no authentic healing internally or externally outside the power, love and compassion of Christ our Lord, our Creator and lover of our souls. Truly no one loves you like Jesus.

C H A P T E R 2

Emotional and Spiritual Detox

The best detox in the world, hands down, is learning to love yourself the way God designed you. If you had or have to explant, healing physically is largely affected by healing spiritually, mentally and emotionally. If you are constantly belittling yourself, there is healing required. If you are constantly trying to better yourself with superficial substances such as heavy make-up, expensive clothing, or body alterations, healing is required. Hating yourself is not only harmful to you but also to those who love you.

Have you ever had a friend who perpetually beats themselves up? It's not only annoying but it is disconcerting that someone would think so little of themselves. We are created in the image of God whether we are aware of this fact or not. Romans 12:1-2 states, "I appeal to you therefore, brothers, by the mercies of God, to present your bodies as a living sacrifice, holy and acceptable to God, which is your spiritual worship. Do not be conformed to this world, but be transformed by the renewal of your mind, that by testing you may discern what is the will of God, what is good and acceptable and perfect."

Personally, I love this text as it gives us, not only encouragement, but instruction. Every issue upon which we find ourselves, the outcome is determined by what is in our minds. Many people who claim to be called by God still do not understand how to get their minds aligned with the righteousness of God. They continuously focus on the natural or, in other words, the things of this earth. Our outer shell, the skin, has been a downfall to countless people throughout the ages; well-meaning people get caught up in outer appearance instead of what matters.

People are busy seeking fame, fortune, approval of people, accolades, and more of the like. All the external things control their every move. Adversely, if these same people would set their minds on things above (heaven), their actions would be very different. They would turn their attentions toward eternal things which are of eternal, long-term value, not just that which brings immediate gratification.

Women especially are dreadfully caught up in our bodies, for the good or bad. We have thousands of movies and TV show which express that beautiful girls or women succeed and the ugly ones fail. We see stick thin girls with enormous breasts, fake tans, fake nails, fake hair, fake eyelashes, and on and on the list goes. There is literally no end to that which is focused on earthly things. God says to get our minds *off* those things and turn our minds toward whatsoever is holy, pure, right, lovely, of good reputation, and all that is excellent (Philippians 4:8). Most of the body of Christ has failed to do just this.

What if you and I began to see ourselves as does God? What if we took our eyes off our bodies and put it on our spirit-man? Imagine a world packed full of women who love themselves (not "in love" with themselves). How would that look? What world-changes would come into effect if that happened? What if we focused on loving God, loving ourselves as is, loving others as they are and living a life of giving rather than seeking that which we can receive? What is we ceased to run after that which would make us sexier, prettier, or more valuable?

This is exactly what needs to happen and God laid the plan within the pages of His holy Word. He knew we would be easily persuaded to follow the world and its corrupted views. He was very aware of the nature of cursed man and gave us a way out. The next chapter will give a plan so as to be able to do just that: love God, love ourselves as is, love mankind and set our minds on things of heaven. It surely will save us a lot of grief and heartache.

Hope, Inspiration and Encouragement

"So we do not lose heart. Though our outer self is wasting away, our inner self is being renewed day by day (II Corinthians 4:16)."

"Just as we have borne the image of the man of dust, we shall also bear the image of the man of heaven (I Corinthians 15:49)."

"Do not lie to one another, seeing that you have put off the old self with its practices and have put on the new self, which is being renewed in knowledge after the image of its Creator (Colossians 3:9-10)."

Regardless of where you are today, there is hope. There is encouragement for the most discouraged. God is in love with you. God created you in His image. He has a plan and a purpose for you just as you are. Whatever pain, suffering and/or trials you are currently experiencing, He has a plan, a great one! God desires to take what Satan means against you for evil and turn it for good. The catch to that promise in Romans 8:28 is to "love the Lord". It reads, "And we know that God causes all things to work together for good *to those who love God, to those who are called according to His purpose.*"

Surrendering your life to Christ is the answer to all your problems. It doesn't mean things will suddenly disappear but it does mean He will usher peace in the worst of chaos. He will begin to open doors which were previously closed to you. He will begin to speak to you and guide you through His Spirit who dwells within you. He earnestly desires for you to know the height, width, length and depth of His irreversible unwavering love and there is nothing greater. His love for you will cause you to fall in love with Him. In such love, the cares and woes of this life will pass to the wayside. In other words, His love will overshadow the problems. He will teach you how to be at peace with the things about yourself you do not like which cannot be changed (or should not be surgically altered).

No, I'm not saying no one should ever have cosmetic surgery as that is a personal decision which could stem from wanting to rectify birth defects to removing unsightly excess skin from massive weight loss to simply not liking a body part and wanting to be more attractive. Regardless, through submission to Christ, the Spirit of God will allow you to see things more clearly; therefore, you will be equipped to make better, more informed and sane decisions *not* based on emotions. One of our more intense enemies in this life is our emotions as they can run amuck on a dime. Through the power of Holy Spirit, He will teach each of us to stop being led around by the nose by feelings and emotions. Nine times out of ten, our emotions are not in alignment with God.

Setting your mind on "things above" may sound simple but it really is a paradigm changer. It will shift your atmosphere by first changing how you see things. That will shift how you respond to situations and then you will be better prepared to go forward in life making better life-altering decisions. God is the answer even when you cannot see it. Understanding the heart and intentions of God will exponentially cause you to reevaluate everything you have ever known. Be of good cheer, the Lord your Creator wants to embrace you in all your sufferings so as to cause you to arise from your depression, sorrow, pain, suffering, trials and tribulations. You are not alone.

I fought this fight on my knees in prayer trusting in the darkest hours that God is still God, that He is in love with me and that He had a good plan for my life. No matter how bleak things appeared and felt in my body, I knew that, through prayer, I would come out eventually. God is not the "quick fix" God, that's who Satan is. Too often we want the immediate fix, but God does not operate on our timeframe. He is steady and steadfast and this requires our patience as He not only works our circumstances out for good, but He carefully and slowly develops good character, patience, perseverance and hope. Every event in life, big and small, is with great purpose so as to lead us into the righteousness of God. Place you faith in the Lord Jesus Christ and watch Him bring all kinds of healing into your life. Be blessed!

"Therefore, having been justified by faith, we have peace with God through our Lord Jesus Christ, through whom also we have obtained our introduction by faith into this grace in which we stand; and we exult in hope of the glory of God. And not only this, but we also exult in our tribulations, knowing that tribulation brings about perseverance; and perseverance, proven character; and proven character, hope; and hope does not disappoint, because the love of God has been poured out within our hearts through the Holy Spirit who was given to us (Romans 5:1-5)."

Closing Prayer

Father, I plead the holy blood of Jesus Christ over each and every reader. First, I pray she finds You, that she will come to know and experience the height, width, length and depth of Your unfailing love. Secondly, I pray that the healing balm of Gilead be poured over her from the top of her head to the soles of her feet. Father, I beseech You to lay Your healing hand upon her body, soul, mind and spirit. Allow her to be guided into all righteousness for Your name's sake. I pray for every demonic spirit of hell to be bound, gagged and loosed from its assignment over her and for Your Spirit to indwell her. I pray for her to recognize what's going on with her body that she may seek and find the right doctor who will aid in her healing. I pray for the money needed for an explant to come from the origin of Your choosing and that You will receive the honor and glory. I ask, Father, for You to bring peace to her, especially in the area of low self-esteem. Where she hates her body, reveal to her in Your goodness that she is fearfully and wonderfully made in Your image. Show her that in her weakest areas, You are more than capable and willing to be her strength. Bring her out of this dark and dreaded place as upon the wings of eagles. Take what Satan meant against her to destroy her and turn it for good as only You can. I pray for the peace which passes all understanding to be as a necklace around her neck and a bracelet around her wrists all the days of her life. Selah.

Written by Alexys V. Wolf

If you have come across this book and it happens you have never been properly introduced to God, this closing is a brief overview of how to come into the kingdom of God through Christ.

Believe:

"He then brought them out and asked, 'Sir, what must I do to be saved?' They replied, '*Believe in the Lord Jesus*, and you will be saved (Acts 16:29).'"

"For John came to you to show you the way of righteousness, and you did not believe him, but the tax collectors and the prostitutes did. And even after you saw this, you did not repent and believe him (Matthew 21:32)."

"For all have sinned and fall short of the glory of God" is found in Romans 3:23. You must believe you dwell in a sinful nature derived from Adam and The Fall of all mankind. Secondly, you must believe that Jesus is Lord; that He gave His life for sinful mankind (you) and accept such a supernatural gift. It is simultaneously the easiest and hardest decision of anyone's life.

In response to such a belief in the Savior, you can take hold of this Scripture: "whosoever shall call on the name of the Lord shall be saved (Acts 2:21)." You are "whosoever." Call out to Him – He's waiting.

Repentance Requirement:

"This is what is written: The Messiah will suffer and rise from the dead on the third day, and *repentance for the forgiveness of sins* will be preached in His name to all nations…(Luke 24:46-47)."

"Jesus answered them, 'It is not the healthy who need a doctor, but the sick. I have not come to call the righteous, but *sinners to repentance* (Luke 5:31-32)."

Repentance is not for God, it's for you. It's an act of absolute humility (also a requirement for the presence of God to rest upon you). Repentance ushers God's grace through such humility.

Baptism to Eternal Life:

"For *you have died* and your life is hidden with Christ in God (Colossians 3:3)."

"I baptize you with water, but He will *baptize you with the Holy Spirit* (Mark 1:8)."

"He who has believed and has been *baptized shall be saved*; but he who has disbelieved shall be condemned (Mark 16:16)."

"Therefore we have been *buried with Him through baptism into death*, so that as Christ was raised from the dead through the glory of the Father, so we too might walk in newness of life (Romans 6:4)."

"For all of you who were baptized into Christ have clothed yourselves with Christ (Galatians 3:27)."

~

This takes belief a step further. Baptism here, contrary to the modern-day church, *precedes* salvation not *succeeds*. This is not physical baptism but spiritual. We are to surrender ourselves unto death in the spiritual sense so as to be able to receive a spiritual new life; hence the Scripture, "I have been crucified in Christ therefore it's no longer I who live but Christ who lives in me (Galatians 2:20)."

Baptism, metaphorically speaking, is the equivalent of crucifixion, aka death to self. We are "buried in His death." When we come to Christ, we must see ourselves as dead so that we can receive His life. Just praying a "sinner's prayer" (which isn't scriptural) is not the same as surrender; surrender is death.

Think about it like this. When one drowns, it's because they can no longer breathe under water; if they could, they'd save their life. When they finally recognize they have no power to rescue themselves, they literally surrender their lives unto the watery death. When we take on Christ's baptism (water of the Word), we must visualize ourselves as "going under"; we are drowning our natural man because we have no power to save ourselves. In the spirit realm, we baptize into death all that came from the bloodline of Adam. In this death condition, we are now available to take His new life; we are regenerated by a new bloodline from Jesus who is of heaven. We take a brand new origin. We are no longer "of the earth" but are "of heaven." This is how we become "strangers in the land of earth."

With this new origin, we are to think from the vantage of our homeland, the kingdom of God. This level of surrender causes a person to stop giving into the temptations of the natural man. This brings us back to understanding we have but one nature while renting space in that of another nature. You are not your flesh or any of it's feelings, desires, or temptations. When tempted with sexual sin such as homosexuality, adultery, pornography, pedophilia or fornication in any form, the flesh wants what it wants, no doubt. However, the surrendered spirit (the real you) within a human shell desires so much to please the One who gave him new and eternal life, he will say 'no' emphatically because he comprehends that life in the flesh is nothing short of despair, anguish, suffering, and destruction.

Drowning in Christ causes the newness and you cannot have newness without first going through such drowning. Many in the modern day church preach 'accept Christ and then be baptized with water immersion.' However, Scriptures would indicate the opposite. We are to believe in the Father and Son unto salvation, be baptized into His Spirit, then water baptism may follow; however, the man on the cross received the kingdom of heaven through faith yet was never water baptized. Unfortunately, we often misrepresent the purpose of baptism as if it's merely by water.

Grace and Repentance:

"Produce fruit in keeping with repentance (Matthew 3:8)."

"Three times I pleaded with the Lord to take it away from me. But He said to me, 'My grace is sufficient for you, for my power is made perfect in weakness.' Therefore I will all the more gladly boast about my weaknesses, so that Christ's power may rest on me (II Corinthians 12:8-9, NAS)."

"For it is by grace you have been saved, through faith – and this is not from yourselves, it is the gift of God, not by works, so that no one can boast (Ephesians 2:8-9, NAS)."

～

Definition of Grace:
1. the free and unmerited favor of God, as manifested in the salvation of sinners and the bestowal of blessings
2. God giving you what you do not deserve (heaven vs. hell; life vs. death; peace vs. chaos)
3. the catalyst for an otherwise impossible transformation from the old man of Adam to the new man in Christ

Definition of Repentance:
1. to turn from sin and dedicate oneself to the amendment of one's life
2. to feel regret or contrition *leading* to change one's mind
3. to cause to feel regret or contrition
4. to feel sorrow, regret, or contrition

Anyone who teaches grace outside repentance and surrender is a false prophet. Surrender and repentance are a requirement so as to receive the grace of God. Yes, we live in the Day of Grace so it is extended to all mankind on a general level, but in respect to walking in personal grace on a regular basis comes through a heart rent before a Holy God. In this condition of perpetual repentance of the sin nature as a whole, His grace is surely sufficient for you and whatever situational crisis you may face.

When I write "perpetual repentance" I mean, simply stated, walking perpetually in an attitude of cosigning all the lusts of the flesh unto God. It's as the Scripture directs, "being ready to punish all disobedience until personal obedience is achieved." An attitude of repentance does *not* mean to self-abase, that is sin (Colossians 2:18, 23). Insulting, belittling, and beating oneself is self-abasement – that is not repentance. Repentance insists that you apologize to God for your action(s), you go and sin no more, and continue unashamed going about the Father's business. In true repentance, you are neither ashamed nor boastful in yourself because self is dead to the world and it's lusts.

Fruit of the Spirit of God can produce only from a place of humility which leads to repentance which leads to grace.

Faith:

"Now faith is confidence in what we hope for and assurance about what we do not see. This is what the ancients were commended for (Hebrews 11:1-2)."

"Without faith it is impossible to please God (Hebrews 11:6)."

"Therefore, since we have been justified by faith, we have peace with God through our Lord Jesus Christ, through whom we have gained access by faith into this grace in which we now stand. And we boast in the hope of the glory of God (Romans 5:1-2)."

Faith is an extension of belief, but stronger than belief alone. Even the demons believe and shutter (James 2:19). Faith says, "I not only believe You exist, but I place all my hope in You" unlike the demons. Faith moves the immovable, touches the untouchable, and makes the impossible possible.

Forgiveness:

"Therefore, my friends, I want you to know that through Jesus the forgiveness of sins is proclaimed to you. Through Him everyone who believes is set free from every sin, a justification you were not able to obtain under the law of Moses (Acts 13:38-39)."

Forgiveness has been extended by God through Jesus to all mankind, whether or not any of us receive it. It was granted to all mankind at the Cross and resurrection of Christ. To receive it, all you must do is repent and it's yours. From there, the rest will come with great ease!

Repent to God, accept His forgiveness. Forgive yourself. Forgive others. Let go of the shame, guilt, remorse, and condemnation; let go of the lies, fear, doubt anxiety as they lead you further and further into darkness.

A New Master!

"For sin shall no longer be your master, because you are not under the law, but under grace (Romans 6:14, NAS)."

"If the Son sets you free, you will be free indeed (John 8:36)."

"But now that you have been *set free from sin* and have become *slaves of God*, the benefit you reap leads to holiness, and the result is eternal life (Romans 6:22)."

"It is for freedom that Christ has set us free. Stand firm, then, and do not let yourselves be burdened again by a yoke of slavery (Galatians 5:1)."

"'I have the right to do anything,' you say – but not everything is beneficial. 'I have the right to do anything' – but I will not be mastered by anything (I Corinthians 6:12)."
"In him and through faith in him we may approach God with freedom and confidence (Ephesians 3:12)."

"You, my brothers and sisters, were called to be free. But do not use your freedom to indulge the flesh; rather, serve one another humbly in love. For the entire law is fulfilled in keeping this one command: 'Love your neighbor as yourself (Galatians 5:13-14).'"

Once you were alienated from God and were enemies in your minds because of your evil behavior. But now He has reconciled you by Christ's physical body through death to present you holy in His sight, without blemish and free from accusation – if you continue in your faith, established and firm, and do not move from the hope held out in the gospel. This is the gospel that you heard and that has been proclaimed to every creature under heaven, and of which I, Paul, have become a servant (Colossians 1:21-23)."

There is no greater gift from God than freedom! There is no greater pleasure or fulfillment in life than serving such a master because this master is like no other. He is Father, Husband, Comforter, Healer, Redeemer, Forgiver – this is a master I can follow through eternity!

By surrendering to such a magnificent, loving, righteous, just, holy God, you will begin to see that jumping from a ledge in order to "end my problems" will no longer appear feasible; it's facade will no longer have the power to overtake you. In Christ, there is no greater place of peace, regardless of the storm, which stems from the liberty found only in knowing and consigning your life to Yahweh. That proverbial ledge will be revealed for what it is – of Satan.

Whatever mess you've concocted, whatever trial besets you, no matter what is happening or for whatever reason, when you submit unto death the nature of the flesh, God commands Himself to take what Satan means against you for evil and turn it for good. I've quoted this Scripture a million times over yet I will continue to do so because many folks still don't get it. In Christ, there is no dilemma, only benefits from His kingdom solution. Every horrible, disastrous, despicable situation is a platform God utilizes to catapult His people onto higher ground.

For more detailed information on this matter, I suggest reading the Bible beginning with the gospels so as to follow the life of Christ, the One who overcame death and the grave and every temptation known to man. He overcame the flesh while living in it. Once He is allowed to take over your life, you too will be able to do as He because His completed work will begin to manifest through you. Additionally, I have written numerous books elaborating on the subjects of knowing your identity in Christ, who you are in the kingdom of God, how to draw closer to the heart of God, and much more.

If you learn nothing else from this, know that God is in love with you and always will be. He formed you in your mother's womb. He allowed your life to be spared thus far. There is life beyond this crisis. There is joy beyond this sorrow. There is acceptance beyond your rejections. There is gain after your loss. There is life outside death. Be encouraged and of good cheer, for Christ is in love with you today!

Author Bio

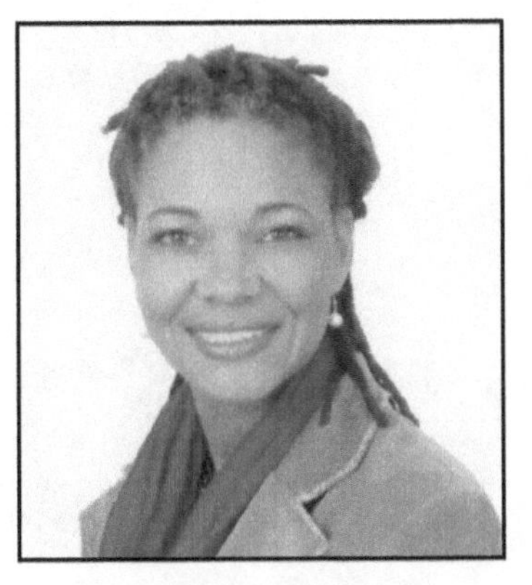

Angelia is a devout Christian who grew up in Seattle Washington. She and her husband and children live in Dallas, Texas. She's been in the dental field for over 25 years. Angelia began writing in 2012 and published her first book, *Fig Leaves* in 2013. Since that time, she has published a children's picture book, *Planting Seeds of Faith*. Angelia is the founder of *Fig Leaves Ministry* which consists of counseling marriages and witnessing to women and children. Her goal is to teach people how to walk according to the Spirit of God in holiness and righteousness. Within that teaching, she instructs females how to dress according to modesty despite the current climate of inappropriate attire peddled at every clothier.

God spared her life and restored her health while battling breast implant illness from 2015-2019. Angelia vowed, even during her sickness, to use her testimony and voice to advocate and educate other women and young girls. God has blessed her and her family tremendously in all areas of life and she is daily paying it forward. Along with her husband, Keith, they founded *TOTB-Dental Staffing Agency* in

2013. She is also the proprietor of *That Cake Lady* which specializes in custom wedding cakes.

If you are interested in inviting Angelia as a guest, please reach out to her at: Angelia.Russell9036@gmail.com

Bibliography

Planting Seeds of Faith, Angelia Russell

Looking for God (3 volumes), Alexys V. Wolf

Casting, Alexys V. Wolf

Walking the Path of Freedom, Alexys V. Wolf

Wise as a Serpent, Innocent as a Dove, Alexys V. Wolf

Talking Yourself off the Ledge, Alexys V. Wolf

When All My Strength Has Failed, Alexys V. Wolf

Navigating the Fiery Black Holes of Life, Alexys V. Wolf

Wielding the Sword of the Spirit. Alexys V. Wolf

Looking for God (3 volumes), Alexys V. Wolf